Better
Sleep,
Better
You

ALSO BY FRANK LIPMAN, MD:

How to Be Well
(with Amely Greeven)

Young and Slim for Life

The New Health Rules
(coauthored with Danielle Claro)

Revive
(with Mollie Doyle)

Total Renewal
(with Stephanie Gunning)

The New Rules of Aging Well

Better
SLEEP,
Better
YOU

FRANK LIPMAN, MD

and

NEIL PARIKH, COFOUNDER OF CASPER

with

RACHEL HOLTZMAN

Thorsons

*For my grandson Benjamin, who reminded me what it's like to
sleep like a baby.*

—Frank

*For our team at Casper, who work tirelessly to awaken the
potential of a well-rested world.*

—Neil

———————

Thorsons
An imprint of HarperCollins*Publishers*
1 London Bridge Street
London SE1 9GF

www.harpercollins.co.uk

HarperCollins*Publishers*
1st Floor, Watermarque Building, Ringsend Road
Dublin 4, Ireland

First published by Thorsons 2021

1 3 5 7 9 10 8 6 4 2

© Frank Lipman, MD & Neil Parikh 2021

Frank Lipman, MD and Neil Parikh asserts the moral right to be
identified as the authors of this work

A catalogue record of this book is available from the British Library

ISBN 978-0-00-839860-6

Illustrations by Giacomo Bagnara

Printed and bound in Great Britain by CPI Group (UK) Ltd, Croydon

CONTENTS

CHAPTER 4
LIVE TO SLEEP

CHAPTER 5
MOVE TO SLEEP

CHAPTER 6
EAT TO SLEEP

CHAPTER 7
SANCTUARY TO SLEEP

CHAPTER 8
SLEEP THROUGH THE AGES

CHAPTER 9
IN YOUR DREAMS

CHAPTER 10
THE RESET

Dependent on sleep are: happiness and misery, nourishment and suitable physique, potency and impotency, knowledge and ignorance. Sleep observed untimely, excessively and negatively takes away happiness and life like the goddess Kalaratri. If properly observed, it provides happiness and life like the flash of true knowledge to a yogini.

— *Charaka Samhita Sutrasthana*

**Better
Sleep,
Better
You**

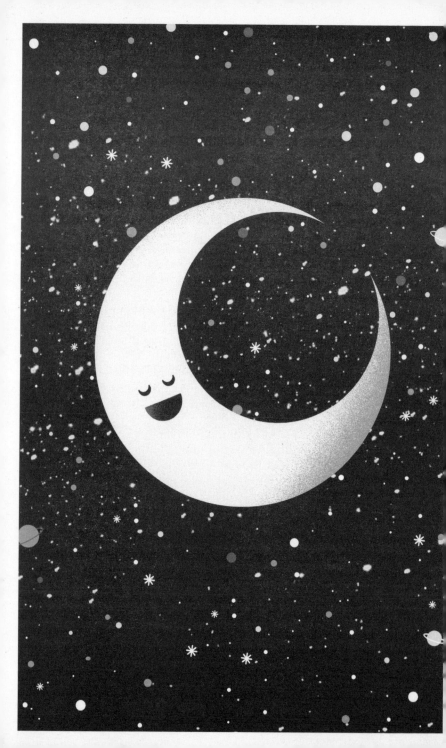

IT'S TIME TO GET COZY WITH SLEEP

You aren't getting enough sleep. Yes, that's a pretty bold statement, since we don't exactly know you, but if you're like most people—and we're willing to bet that you are—then you're not getting the rest you need. The numbers alone do the talking: 40 percent of Americans report occasional insomnia, 22 percent experience insomnia almost every night, and *70 percent* of Americans aren't getting enough sleep, no thanks to shifts in our culture (twenty-four-hour everything), technology (all Wi-Fi, all the time), and habits (overworking, under-nourishing). Unfortunately, the seemingly small oversight of not get-ting enough sleep—whether it's because you're choosing other priorities over sleep or you're having sleep-related challenges that don't seem to be going away anytime soon—will most likely end up having some very big consequences, if it hasn't already. But not to worry; that's all about to change. Namely because you're about to read the very first one-stop sleep-better resource that's perfectly tailored to you, your sleep, and your life.

From the time we, the authors, first met, we knew that we were going to team up to improve people's lives. In fact, that's why we were introduced in the first place—because a mutual friend knew how obsessed we each were with that mission. Neil first came to Frank as a patient—he wanted a new approach to feeling better and liked Frank's holistic philosophy (as in, better sleep leads to improvement in your overall health, and improvement in your overall health leads to better sleep) along with his tough-love style (a little bit of a whooping followed by a carrot). Meanwhile, Frank was inspired by Neil's passion for the emerging tools and technologies that help form new, better habits, especially when it comes to getting a good night's rest. After weeks of daily e-mails back and forth about our respective discoveries of new gadgets, therapies, and ideas around sleep and behavior change, this book was born. Our mission: Write a book that would finally get people in bed to get the rest they need.

Especially in the wake of Covid-19, when even more people began struggling with maintaining healthy sleep habits and it became clear that lack of sleep was a comorbidity in the virus, we knew that we needed to do something different from what had already been done. Most of you have seen the articles (or at least read the headlines). You already know that we are currently experiencing a sleep-deprivation epidemic, and you're aware—either anecdotally or firsthand—that most people are paying the price. From an out-of-whack immune system, to weight gain, to hormone dysregulation, to brain chemistry imbalance, or even worse, heart disease, diabetes, and Alzheimer's, you're at least somewhat aware of the price you pay when you don't get enough sleep. And on the flip side, tons of studies have confirmed that if we just get more sleep—more than the five or six hours we've been telling ourselves is plenty—then we can fend off both major and minor illnesses, boost our ability to learn, solve problems better, think outside the box, lose weight, look and feel younger, and better manage stress. Plus, there's no shortage of clickbait articles outlining just about every sound piece of advice for sleeping more or better, whether it's unplugging from our devices an hour before bedtime, using room-darkening shades, or taking a lavender oil–infused bath before bed.

And yet, we are all still exhausted.

Not many people sleep any better than we did before the emerging research gave us an even clearer understanding of why sleep is so important, what it does for every single element of our health, and how to get more of it. So to everyone walking around feeling like they're living in a fog, like they're moving at half speed, like they can't shake their depression/anxiety, and like they, perhaps, may never get a good night's sleep ever again, this book is for you. It's also for those of you who aren't quite there but feel irritable, dulled, worn out, and worn down. We have made it our goal to figure out why it's so difficult to do anything about it—and to fix it.

We believe the fix begins with changing the way you think about sleep. For the longest time, the three big pillars of wellness have been diet, exercise, and stress. Important, yes, but not the whole picture. Without adequate sleep, a healthy diet, regular exercise, and stress management aren't enough to comprehensively transform or even maintain your health. That's because **sleep is your primary rhythm**. Every single system of your body is regulated by your circadian rhythm, which is your body's own 24-hour rhythm that synchronizes your cardiovascular, muscular, digestive, immune, and reproductive systems. But the queen of these individual rhythms is sleep. That's why we like to say *sleep is your primary rhythm*: **all roads lead to and from sleep.** When sleep is off, so is every other function in your body. Think of it this way:

1. If you're trying to solve a health-related issue but are not addressing sleep, then you're swimming against the current.
2. Or, if you're experiencing sleep-related issues, that could likely be a symptom that something is off in another system of your physiology. (It can also, though, just be a sleep issue.)

3. However, if you remedy your sleep by taking steps to address all the facets of your health that feed sleep, those benefits flow downstream to enrich every element of your wellness.

In other words, **the key to living a longer, healthier life often starts with focusing on sleep. And the road back to bed is paved with getting back into rhythm.**

To help you get there, we've developed a simple yet powerful approach: Making a series of small shifts in your daily habits, all in the name of resetting your body's natural clock. For the first time, you will be able to clearly understand your unique rhythms and sleep needs, then curate the ideal regimen that's perfectly tailored to your body, physiology, and lifestyle. And to help you see quick, promising results, we've also included The Reset—a quick, (relatively) painless, whole-system refresh. By essentially pushing the restart button on your internal clock, you'll immediately see the positive association between the choices you make and your sleep.

Ultimately, this guide is yours to take with you for the rest of your life. It is here to help you navigate your own evolving sleep needs, as well as those of your children and parents (check out "Sleep Through the Ages" on page 204—it will likely surprise you). This book is here for you to revisit when you need the occasional rhythm reset or you encounter an issue—like sleep apnea, jet lag, or having a newborn—that needs troubleshooting. By developing and sticking to your own sleep protocol, you'll be taking important steps toward not only improving your sleep health, but also eating better, functioning better, and chilling out more. And as a result, you'll be unlocking a (long) lifetime of dynamic energy, boundless creativity, resilient wellness, and of course, many, many sweet dreams.

MEET YOUR SLEEP-BETTER SUPPORT TEAM

We both like to think of ourselves as professionals in making people's lives a little bit easier, a little bit healthier, and certainly more enjoyable.

For Frank, a doctor of functional and integrative medicine, that's meant over forty years of offering his clients powerful, simple habit changes as a prescription versus popping a pill (and another and another). Instead of medicating away the symptoms, these shifts put his patients in touch with their natural rhythms, which in turn addresses the underlying cause of their symptoms. With a background in traditional Chinese medicine (TCM) as well, Frank's approach to treating patients is less like that of a mechanic and more like that of a gardener. The mechanic-like Western-medicine MO is typically to find the broken part, then fix it (medicate it) or remove it (operate on it). Whereas in TCM, the goal is for the patient, like a plant, to flourish and grow. If the leaves are turning yellow, you don't just remove them or paint them green—you look to see if the roots are being impinged, if the soil is nutrient-rich enough, if the plant is getting enough sun, water, etc. It's looking at the underlying issues that are resulting in the problem. Now he's turning his attention to sleep as both the symptom *and* a root cause of sub-optimal health. And as a member of the Casper Sleep Advisory Board, he's helping many more frustrated sleepers—in addition to the Casper staff—get the sleep education they want and need to make their lives even better.

His sleep superpowers: Giving you all the information you need (including up-to-the-minute studies and research) but in a way that doesn't require a medical degree to understand, along with a doctor-approved protocol for how to feel better *right now.*

Neil is the son of a sleep doctor and the cofounder of Casper, a company focused on revolutionizing how people think about sleep and invest in their nighttime habits. His mission has been to give people some of the most important tools for making life better, from pillows that eliminate aches and pains, to lamps that automatically dim and encourage your body's wind-down response, to mattresses, which should be to sleep what Nikes are to running—they should make you feel like you could conquer the world! He and his team are also at the forefront of creating a culture where sleep can seem like less of a have-to and more of a can't-wait-to. In addition to creating the Casper Sleep Advisory Board, which is made up of some of the most prominent experts on wellness and sleep (including Frank) and advises the team and Casper customers on the latest innovations and theories regarding superior z's, the Casper team also walks the walk. They are the front-line guinea pigs putting their gear and recommendations to the test, making sure that what they're offering actually works. In fact, they were the first subjects for The Reset, which you'll learn more about in Chapter 10.

And maybe most important, Neil has been where you are! His need to address his own sleep issues (namely still feeling exhausted, even after a seemingly full night's sleep) is what ultimately brought him to Frank. Together, they examined Neil's habits: too much caffeine during the day and too late in the afternoon, late meals owing to work or social outings, unpredictable sleep and wake times, and way too much stress. The result was basically ongoing jet lag, or as Frank described it, being "out of rhythm." To get back into rhythm, Neil had to reassess which habits were actively stealing from his sleep (all that caffeine, late-night meals and snacking, not managing his stress, variable bedtimes, falling asleep in front of the TV) and to adopt more beneficial behaviors (switching to half-caf Americanos, yoga, meditation, moving the TV out of his room, adding supplements like CBD and magnesium). He had to look at his exercise, his diet, and his lifestyle in a whole new way in order to understand the 24-hour cycle of sleep. The stress didn't magically disappear, and his evening obligations couldn't always be rescheduled, but what he could change, he did. The result? Better sleep!

His sleep superpowers: Using his expansive knowledge about the latest gear and gadgets to help you get a better night's sleep, along with a been-there-done-that sensibility from someone who's been in the trenches of less-than-stellar sleep.

TIME FOR SOME REAL TALK

If you're going to unlock the next-level health-enhancing, life-lengthening, all-around-optimizing benefits of sleep, then you're going to have to start treating a good night's rest like it matters. Because it does—*a lot*. And nothing illustrates the incredible power of sleep more starkly than seeing what happens when you don't get enough. Sleep deprivation, which kicks in after even just one night of getting less than you need, affects every single one of your major organ systems, from your heart to your brain to your immune system. It negatively impacts how well you learn, how clearly you think, how gracefully you age, how well you fend off illness, your mood, your ability to get in the mood, and your weight. Sleep deprivation is a proven risk factor for Alzheimer's, cancer, heart disease, heart attack/failure, stroke, diabetes, depression, anxiety, and obesity.

In fact, not getting enough sleep can harm your very DNA, the blueprint from which everything in your body is made. Researchers observed in sleep-deprived study participants that their DNA produced fewer "repair genes" and more DNA "breaks." That means that they had fewer genes that can correct potentially harmful mutations as cells in the body duplicate, as well as more damage in the DNA. This is further evidence that lack of quality sleep is a contributing factor to cancer as well as cardiovascular, metabolic, and neurodegenerative diseases.[1]

Sleep really is a matter of life and death. In a 2007 study, British researchers revealed how sleep patterns affected their 10,000 subjects, whom they had observed over twenty years. The results were clear: Those who skimped on sleep nearly doubled their risk of death from all causes (though particularly cardiovascular disease).[2] And not to pile on, but according to new research published by the *Journal of the American Heart Association,* if you're already dealing with chronic disease like high blood pressure, type 2 diabetes, heart disease, or stroke, then you're at an even higher risk for cancer and early death if you're not getting sufficient sleep.[3]

So let's just all agree on one thing: **Better sleep = a better life.**

LEARNING HOW TO SLEEP BETTER DOESN'T HAVE TO BE A SNOOZE

Thanks to the feedback we've gotten from our patients, clients, coworkers, friends, and family, we've dedicated this book to *simplicity*—because no one wants or needs another dense, complicated, research-heavy book about sleep. (Though, we'd argue that trying to read said book could be a potential sleep-inducing solution . . .) But seriously, getting better sleep shouldn't be boring. And it definitely shouldn't be difficult. Though, it made us wonder: If sleep's so important, why aren't more people getting the rest they need? The way we see it, there's a few things standing in the way:

- **There's a ton of information out there—and it's not exactly bedtime reading.** It's overwhelming and it's difficult to understand. Plus, what's the last thing you want to do when you're exhausted and not functioning optimally? Slog through dense chapters full of scientific research. It's fascinating and important, but we think the information you need to start feeling better should be distilled into highly digestible, compulsively readable, and bite-sized pieces accompanied by usable, actionable advice. Will we include some research? Yes. Will it require you to put down your phone for a minute and pay attention? Yes. But do we promise to keep it short and sweet? Absolutely.

■ **Sleep has become a chore.** It's yet another thing on the seemingly endless list of things you "should" be doing to feel better. Instead of being part of a natural rhythm that you seamlessly drift into at the end of the day, it feels like something that is being wedged in between work obligations, kids' bedtime routines, and social engagements. So you figure, "Why not just pop a pill?" That, unfortunately, not only negatively affects your overall health but also damages your sleep wellness in the longterm. We want you to feel like you *get* to sleep. When the body's natural rhythms are reset— meaning you're eating, moving, and living in a way that supports the cycles that govern sleep all day long (something we'll be talking about *much* more in a bit)—sleep will come easily and naturally.

■ **It's tough to know which new habits will work best for you—or how to gauge if they're working.** If you want to learn how to exercise in a way that works best for your body, health needs, and personal interests, you can hire a personal trainer. If you want to adopt a new way of eating that is both impactful and realistic for your life, you can hire a nutritionist. But for sleep, most experts still apply too wide a range of advice to too wide a range of people. Your own unique sleep protocol should be a reflection of your unique rhythm, taking into account your age, physiology, lifestyle, and preferences. And just like with fitness, there are now tools to actively track sleep as a metric.

- **You don't want to give up the things you enjoy.** If it were easy to live like monks in the name of getting better sleep, everyone would be doing it. But that's just not how the world works. No one wants to commit to a life full of restrictions. That's why we have developed a program that's tailored to your own preferences and needs—social life and guilty pleasures included. Then, by monitoring your own progress using sleep-tracking methodology or a good old-fashioned pen-and-paper sleep log, you'll be able to see how the choices you make throughout the day either help or hurt your sleep patterns—so *you* can ultimately make the best choices for yourself, not us. And know how to get back on track when you fall off the wagon.

- **There is no one–sleep–fits–all solution.** "Tell me how to sleep!" is one of the most common pleas Frank hears in his practice. And yet, in all of his forty years as a doctor he has confirmed, by treating thousands of patients with varying degrees and types of sleep deprivation, that there is no one single, universal recommendation. And that's because of a few things:

  1. There's not one "perfect" amount of sleep.
  2. Each of our bodies is different.
  3. There are a number of lifestyle factors that affect our sleep, and they don't just occur at night.

But while there may not be one universal solution, there is one frequent cause of not-great sleep: That's right, being out of rhythm. So in this book we'll be walking you through each of the factors that may be throwing you out of rhythm, including when and what you eat, how and when you move, how you handle stress, and how and when you nap. We'll also be looking at all the physiological factors that influence rhythm—things like your age, gut health, hormones, and even genes can make a difference. Your ideal sleep protocol will most likely look different than your partner's, your parents', or even your peers'—and that's normal. By helping you figure out how to listen to your own body and examine your existing habits, we'll help you figure out the right amount of sleep for you and the best way to get there—backed by your own individual results.

CHAPTER I

GETTING IN RHYTHM WITH REST

We have gotten very good at believing that we get to make our own rhythms, independent from nature's. We live a fast-paced, 24-7 lifestyle (usually indoors under artificial lighting) before trying to go to sleep at whatever hour we can (usually too late and with more artificial lighting from screens, LED and fluorescent lights, etc.). We work long hours, never getting a break from our in-boxes, newsfeeds, phone calls, and virtual meetings, and we are constantly juggling obligations to our children, friends, and family, all the while being bombarded by other stressors. We are under-slept and overtired, and when we wake up in the morning, the cycle begins again. If we burn out, no biggie—there's a drug for that. Same goes for any health side effects we may experience, such as energy slumps, blood pressure spikes, hormonal imbalance, mood swings, decreased libido, or increased anxiety and depression. Our lives don't seem so abnormal because everyone around us is living the exact same way and experiencing the same symptoms.

What we all have in common, and what Frank sees in almost every single one of his patients, is that *we are sorely out of sync with our environment*. We are out of rhythm. It's what we call **cultural arrhythmia**. And in order to solve your sleep issues—in addition to virtually all your other health-related concerns—we need to remedy that.

Think about the last time you experienced jet lag—and how much it sucks (medically speaking, of course). You get tired easily, feel sluggish, and struggle to concentrate or think clearly. Your body aches, you have trouble sleeping, and you may even have digestive issues. Unfortunately, this phenomenon isn't isolated to far-flung travel. Many of us are putting these rhythms to the test every single day and feeling as though we constantly have jet lag.

In daily life, we fall out of sync because we consistently give our bodies the wrong cues by:

- paying more attention to the clocks on our phones than the clocks in our bodies
- eating the wrong foods at the wrong times
- ingesting rhythm-altering substances (like caffeine, nicotine, and alcohol)
- exercising at the wrong times (or not at all)
- being perpetually stressed
- not spending enough time just relaxing
- not getting enough natural light during the day
- getting too much artificial light around the clock
- not having consistent daily habits (especially not going to sleep and waking up at the same time, including the weekends)
- getting too little or poor sleep (shocker, we know)

All of this adds up to disrupted sleep patterns. And when your sleep is off, so are the rest of your body's functions. That's why there's more to getting the rest you need than simply going to bed earlier or waking up later.

RHYTHM IN THE TIME OF PANDEMIC

The Covid-19 pandemic has been a profound rhythm disruptor for billions of people. Due to our experiences of dramatic shifts in schedule, working from home, job loss, looking after children or other family members all day, social isolation, emotional disturbance, and significant amounts of stress will send long-lasting shockwaves through our sleep-wake patterns and sleep hygiene. The recommendations in this book are well suited to help you recognize and navigate these shifts in your life. We also recommend checking out a free app called Social Rhythms, which was created by scientists at the University of Michigan. This tracking software not only helps the scientists collect more data about how our biological clocks have responded to lockdown, but it also allows users to see their own sleep-wake patterns emerge. We'll talk more about how tracking can be an enormous sleep-better tool on page 50 ("Tracking Your Progress with Sleep Tech"), but suffice it to say that as big fans of data, we think the more information you can collect about your sleep habits, the better.

DOES YOUR RHYTHM NEED A RESET?

If you answer yes to three or more of the questions below, your body is most likely asking to be resynchronized with its most natural rhythms, beginning with sleep:

- Do you wake up in the morning and not feel refreshed?
- Do you feel unusually tired most of the time?
- Do you need coffee, soda, or sugary snacks to get going and keep going?
- Although you feel physically exhausted, does your mind continue to race?

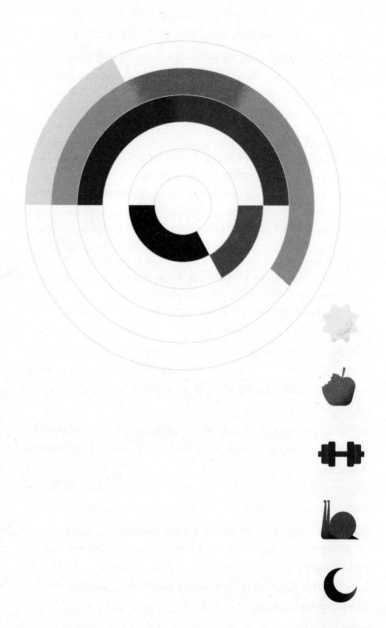

- Do you feel as if you are aging too quickly?
- Do you have gas, bloating, constipation, and/or indigestion?
- Is it a struggle to lose weight in spite of eating well and exercising?
- Do you have achy muscles and/or joints or tension in your body—particularly your neck and shoulders?
- Do you have a diminished sex drive?
- Do you often feel depressed or have trouble concentrating, focusing, and remembering things?
- Have you found that little or nothing seems to rejuvenate you?
- Do you lack motivation to accomplish even small tasks?
- Do you find that you get sick more frequently and that it takes longer to recover?

DAY AND NIGHT: THE RHYTHM MAKERS

The path to a good night's rest begins with this basic understanding: *There are fundamental biological laws that are bigger than you, more pressing than social obligations and work responsibilities, and more powerful than advancements in Western medicine.*

These biological laws were written way back when our ancestors were living in caves and huts, waking with the sun, exerting themselves in spurts, eating what was growing seasonally, and resting as the sky grew dark. Our lives may have changed, but our DNA has not. So when you don't follow these laws, your body will become confused, dysfunctional, and ultimately sick.

These biological "rules" are governed by your **Master Clock**, which is sometimes referred to as your "sleep-wake cycle." The Master Clock's scientific name is the **suprachiasmatic nucleus (SCN)**, which resides at the base of the brain in the hypothalamus. All you need to know is that the Master Clock is an all-powerful internal gauge that coordinates your **circadian rhythms**. These are the physical, mental, and behavioral changes in your body that follow a daily cycle.

So the rhythms dictated by your Master Clock tell your body

when to sleep
when to wake up
when to eat
when to exert

The Master Clock is essentially a pacemaker for the body, coordinating all your systems on a continuous twenty-four-hour loop. To do this, it uses information from your environment in order to sync up with it. And the primary piece of information it uses to do this? Light. Because your body was originally programmed to sleep when it's dark and to be awake when it's light.

Using information from light-detecting cells in your eyes (even when they're closed!), the Master Clock is constantly monitoring the duration and brightness of light—day and night. Depending on this feedback, the Master Clock uses hormones and neurotransmitters (chemical messengers) to cue rhythms throughout the body.

Here's how it looks:

- At first light, the Master Clock taps all the functions that get us going for the day: our hormones rev up to stimulate our metabolism, our body temperature rises, our muscles are primed for movement, and our brain function clicks into focus.
- As darkness falls, the Master Clock prepares us for sleep: the body cools down, digestion enters rest-and-repair mode, and the brain begins its nightly detox regimen, clearing out all of the by-products produced during the day from an active mind, as well as consolidating and storing memories.

Sleep Is Not Just a Nighttime Activity

Looking at the entire 24-hour circadian cycle raises a crucial point about sleep and rhythm: Sleep wellness is not just about what you do at night. While, yes, your nighttime behaviors do make a big difference in how well you sleep, getting back into rhythm means tending to your habits throughout the day. Your Master Clock is continuously running, continuously taking in information, and continuously and cumulatively calibrating. An action that throws off your rhythm at one point in the day is going to cause a domino effect throughout the other smaller rhythms that eventually throws off the entire cycle. That's why the new sleep-strengthening habits we'll be introducing are meant to be incorporated all day long. We know which times of day are best for supporting things like digestion, focus, and exertion, so we'll include a key for which time of day is best for plugging in those new habits. As you begin to properly support your body's functions on a twenty-four-hour basis, you'll see a clear improvement in your sleep and overall wellness.

Your Master Clock oversees more than 100 different circadian rhythms, or twenty-four-hour cycles, throughout your body. For example: the cycle in your gut regulates hunger and digestion, the cycle in your brain controls mental alertness and mood, and the cycle in your lungs affects your breathing. Blood pressure, body temperature, hormone levels, heart rate — every function of your body down to the cellular level has its own unique rhythm, but they are all managed (directly and indirectly) by the Master Clock. And these functions, including sleep, need to be kept in sync in order to achieve optimal wellness.

Each of these different functions peak at different times of the day so that they can perform optimally without overwhelming the body. This is why at certain windows throughout the day your body performs or feels differently. Between 10 a.m. and 12 p.m. you may feel better able to focus or have more energy for a workout, but between 2 p.m. and 4 p.m. you might be ready for a nap. There is, like all things that nature has programmed, a logical rhythm to this delicate ebb and flow — and you can connect to it once again. As you clear out the "noise" of being out of rhythm, you'll be able to tune in to what your body needs and when, whether it's a meal, a jog, a mind-clearing break, or a short rest.

MELATONIN AND CORTISOL: THE RHYTHM KEEPERS

At the center of our sleep-wake choreography are two major players: the hormones and chemical messengers **melatonin** and **cortisol**.

As daylight begins to dim and your Master Clock detects the decrease in light, it increases the production of **melatonin**. This hormone is nature's sleep aid. And by that we're talking about the pure stuff, not the manufactured kind which we'll talk more about on page 166 ("Melatonin: Make It, Don't Fake It"). In a perfect, well-rested world, the production of melatonin would cue you to start winding down and head to bed.

When melatonin levels in your body rise, **cortisol** begins to recede. Cortisol is melatonin's daytime counterpart, promoting alertness, boosting energy, regulating blood pressure, aiding digestion, and increasing blood sugar (actually a good thing in moderation). However, cortisol is also your body's main stress hormone and is released whenever your brain perceives stress—whether it's an actual threat, like getting sick or the effects of global warming, or what we perceive as threats on a daily basis, like work-related e-mail or congested traffic. So you can probably see why increased stress—and therefore cortisol— has such a damaging effect on your sleep, and by extension, your health. But more on that later.

As your cortisol levels (ideally) dip, your energy levels also begin to slow. Once it's fully dark, your body consistently and rhythmically secretes more melatonin with the goal of keeping you asleep so your body can conduct its crucial nightly refresh and repair. Your body needs this time to perform functions like flush and detox the brain, consolidate memories and information, decrease blood pressure, and make more immune cells, which is why melatonin does much more than act as a simple sleep cue. It's also a necessary conductor, coordinating important metabolic functions and keeping your rhythm train running on time.

Then, as the sky brightens in the morning, light-sensor cells detect light from the sun, melatonin secretion stops, and cortisol begins rising once again to get you moving for the day.

WHAT'S MESSING WITH YOUR MELATONIN?

Unfortunately, your Master Clock can be fooled into thinking it's not the right time to release melatonin or into not secreting enough. In fact, because of our modern lifestyles, most of us are guilty of tampering with our biological clocks, with the result being bodies that don't know when to go to bed. When that happens, you have a recipe for a sleep-wake cycle that is chronically out of whack. The most common ways we do this are:

- **Too much artificial light:** Electricity wasn't exactly around yet when your body's blueprint was invented, so it makes sense that your Master Clock hasn't gotten the memo that artificial light from light bulbs and device screens does not equal sunlight. Since your brain still believes that light=day, exposing your Master Clock to too much artificial light is the number one way that people throw off their sleep-wake cycle, making overall sleep time shorter and/or harder to come by.
- **Too little natural light:** If you're not exposed to natural sunlight during the day — which, sadly, most of us aren't as a result of office buildings or bedrooms-turned-offices — that, too, is going to throw off the rhythmic secretions of melatonin, because the sun is what helps our Master Clock synchronize to the day-night cycle.
- **Too much cortisol:** As we mentioned earlier, if your body is secreting more cortisol than is optimal — because of things like unrelenting stress, eating a diet high in sugar, or even exercising too late in the evening — then it starts to affect the delicate waltz between melatonin and cortisol production.
- **Too little consistency:** Your Master Clock was made to call the shots. So if you're overriding the system by eating meals at irregular times and, even more detrimentally, going to bed at irregular times — a phenomenon known as social jet lag, which we'll be spending a lot of time on in a bit — then you are single-handedly messing with the rhythm that nature intended, and as a result, your melatonin production won't be able to keep up.

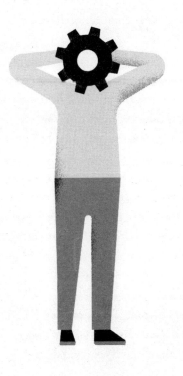

THE OUT-OF-RHYTHM BODY

When your rhythm is off, your entire body knows it. Every single system starts to suffer. Once your sleep is knocked off-kilter, it's not only *creating* an out-of-rhythm effect on your body, it's also an *indication* that something else in your body isn't functioning properly—a cause and a symptom. As sleep dysfunction persists, the dysfunction in your body will only get worse, continuing the cycle.

Mind

The brain is usually the first of your bits to speak up if you're out of rhythm—it's why you feel foggy and sluggish after even just one crummy night's sleep. That's because the brain has a lot of important self-care to catch up on when you've shut down for the night.

It uses that time to forge pathways between nerve cells, helping you retain information that you've learned that day. But if the brain is being taxed doing other things at night (like helping you binge watch Netflix) when it should be refreshing and rebooting, then over time it becomes more difficult for you to focus and learn new things. Sleep deprivation also increases levels of the stress hormone cortisol, which decreases the number of new brain cells that are created in your hippocampus, the brain's learning and memory center. Not getting sufficient sleep also decreases your coordination and increases your risk for accidents and injury. The effects on the brain from sleep deprivation are in many ways similar to the effects of drinking too much alcohol. Some of the latest research shows that drivers who slept even one hour less than they typically do are at significantly higher risk for motor-vehicle crashes.[4] According to the National Sleep Foundation, highly sleep-deprived workers are 70 percent more likely to be in work-related accidents than well-rested workers.[5] And a lack of sleep is linked to a higher risk of injury in athletes,[6] including teenage athletes,[7] who are particularly prone to sleep deprivation, as we'll talk about more in Chapter 8.

The brain also has a nightly detox regimen to tend to, which lack of sleep can inhibit. Just as your muscles generate lactic acid after a workout (essentially the toxic by-product of exercise), the brain also generates damaging proteins over the course of a long day metabolizing all the articles you've read, e-mails you've written, and decisions you've made. And just like sore muscles need to rest and restore, so does your brain. Sleep is meant to be the time that the brain can flush itself of those toxic metabolites, using its own cleansing mechanism called the glymphatic system to rid the brain of harmful proteins. Without sufficient sleep, these proteins begin to accumulate. They form plaque (in the case of amyloid beta protein) and tangles (in the case of tau protein). This leads to cognitive decline and possibly paves the way for Alzheimer's, in addition to contributing to more (disease-causing) sleep disruption.

Researchers at the Washington University School of Medicine in St. Louis have recently reported that subjects who had less slow-wave sleep—the deep sleep you need to consolidate memories and wake up feeling refreshed—had higher levels and more pervasive spread of tau. That's why it's important to focus not just on quantity of sleep, but quality—something we'll help you address.

The sleep you get now also sets up how your brain functions later. In the case of plaque buildup, it can take up to two decades to see symptoms like memory loss and confusion.

Mood

People who are sleep deprived experience an increase in negative moods (anger, frustration, irritability, sadness) and a decrease in positive ones (optimism, levity, easy-goingness). That's because deep sleep is a powerful form of therapy that soothes and balances the brain and, as a result, our emotions. When we shortchange that process, we feel the results. A study from the University of California at Berkeley examined the effects of just one night's loss of sleep, and in looking at the brain scans of otherwise healthy adults, researchers saw that there was more activity in their amygdala—the brain center of fear and anxiety—with participants reporting a noticeable uptick in anxious feelings.[8] A Sleep in America poll found that people diagnosed with depression or anxiety were more likely to sleep less than six hours at night. It's also not a coincidence that those with insomnia are five times as likely to develop depression. Sleep deprivation also leaves you more prone to mood swings and triggers mania in people who have bipolar disorder. And, as researchers at Iowa State University found, sleep loss—even just losing a couple of hours one night—uniquely exacerbates the anger response,[9] making it more difficult to cope with even mildly irritating events.

UC Berkeley researchers have also found that sleep-deprived people feel lonelier and are more inclined to avoid close contact with others, similar to people with social anxiety. As a result, they become less socially attractive to others, to the point where even well-rested people feel lonely after an interaction with a sleep-deprived person. So it's not really exaggerating to say that your lack of sleep is bumming everyone out.[10]

Heart

The American Heart Association is now recommending that doctors look at sleep in addition to other behaviors like diet, exercise, blood pressure, and blood sugar as primary indications of whether a patient is at risk for heart disease. That's because insufficient and poor-quality sleep is linked to a higher risk for heart disease and major heart disease contributors like obesity, type 2 diabetes, and high blood pressure.

Part of the body's upkeep while we sleep includes the production of white blood cells, which the immune system dispatches to fight infection and protect the body from foreign invaders. Because of these cells' aggressive nature and how they battle these invaders, white blood cells are a big source of inflammation in the body. And when deployed more than necessary, they can do more harm than good, including contributing to atherosclerosis, a condition where arteries become hard and inflamed in response to the buildup of plaque.

We do have some control over just how many white blood cells are set loose as a result of sleep, which helps the body regulate the production of inflammatory cells as well as protect the health of its blood vessels. However, as researchers at Massachusetts General Hospital recently found, when we don't get enough sleep, we lose control of inflammatory cell production, leading to more inflammation.[11]

Meanwhile, next door at Harvard, scientists witnessed how white blood cells in a sleep-deprived mouse body essentially get tangled up in arterial plaque, making the existing plaque buildup bigger and more obtrusive. This causes artery-clogging blood clots and reduces blood flow, which in turn sets the stage for heart disease and, over time, heart attacks and strokes. Researchers also discovered that poor sleep reduces the body's levels of hypocretin, a protein that is produced by the hypothalamus—the part of the brain that regulates sleep. The less hypocretin released, the more white blood cells your body generates, and the more likely those cells are to get caught in the plaque that blocks the arteries that causes atherosclerosis, yada yada yada. But on a brighter note, when the team at Harvard gave their sleep-deprived mice supplements of hypocretin—to simulate the aftermath of some much-needed sleep—their atherosclerosis decreased.[12]

Sleep is also a natural blood pressure medication, gently decreasing the inevitably elevated blood pressure you experience from a day's worth of physical and emotional stressors (aka living your life). Without a nightly reset, however, your blood pressure will steadily rise, putting you—once again—at risk for heart attack, stroke, and heart disease. Consider this: On the Monday after we set the clocks forward for daylight savings time in the spring, when we lose an hour of sleep, there's a 25 percent increase in heart attacks worldwide. Compare that to the fall, when we gain an extra hour and there's a 21 percent decrease in heart attacks.[13]

It's also worth noting that adults older than 45 years old with irregular sleeping patterns (no regular bedtime and wakeup schedule, varying amounts of sleep each night) are nearly twice as likely to develop cardiovascular disease as those with regular sleep patterns.[14]

Sex

We'll make this one a quickie: Less sleep means less testosterone in men and in women, which leads to less interest in sex, less pleasurable and frequent sex, erectile dysfunction, and significantly smaller testicles (in men who sleep five hours or fewer a night versus those who sleep eight or more). These same men tend to have the levels of testosterone similar to men ten years older. That's because a small amount of bad sleep—even just one week's worth—is enough to age you a decade when it comes to testosterone production. There's also research showing that sleeping too little may reduce men's fertility.[15] And while there has been shockingly little research done on the effect of sleep deficit on women's fertility, it's safe to say that because of the harmful effects of sleep deprivation on health in general, it most likely does negatively impact your ability to conceive.

Weight

There's a reason it's called "fat and tired": not getting enough sleep is directly linked to gaining weight. Researchers at the University of Colorado found that just one week of sleeping five hours a night resulted in participants gaining an average of two pounds without changing anything else in their diet or exercise regimen. This is because sleep deprivation causes a cascade of changes in your body that leads to weight gain.

First, there's a shift in your hunger-related hormones, including leptin, which suppresses appetite, and ghrelin, which promotes it. Sleep deprivation reduces leptin and increases ghrelin, making you feel hungrier and less satisfied, in addition to changing what kind of food you crave—which, you can probably guess, is not leafy greens. Instead, when you're sleep-deprived, you'll find yourself fixating on foods that are high in sugar and unhealthy fats, which is a result of two changes in your brain that occur when you don't sleep enough. There's the inhibited activity of the frontal lobe (responsible for complex decision-making), in addition to the increased activity in deeper brain centers, which respond to rewards (particularly of the fatty and sugary variety).[16]

Second, bad sleep is bad for gut health. Sleep and circadian disruption can alter your microbiome, the command center in your digestive system that not only breaks down food, but also manufactures hormones and houses a large piece of your immune system. Studies show that disruption to your gut microbiota, or the beneficial bacteria that are supposed to thrive there, is directly linked to weight gain, in addition to a wide range of other health issues, including autoimmune conditions like rheumatoid arthritis, diabetes, chronic fatigue, depression, and insomnia.

Third, sleep deprivation causes the pancreas to release insulin, which leads to increased fat storage and a higher risk of type 2 diabetes.

And fourth, while it's not exactly the most mind-blowing scientific fact, a lack of sleep can make you feel too tired to exercise, which we all know can be an important part of maintaining your ideal weight. These factors combined explain why, according to researchers studying the link between sleep deprivation and weight gain, people who sleep fewer than six hours a day are almost 30 percent more likely to become obese than those who sleep seven to nine hours.[17]

Aging

It's apt that looking "tired" is essentially code for looking old: chronic sleep loss is speeding up your biological clock, and it shows up on your

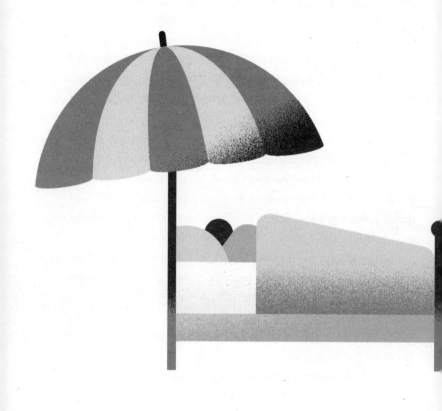

face. Lackluster skin, fine lines, and dark circles under your eyes are all a result of sleep deprivation. When you don't get enough sleep, your body releases more of the stress hormone cortisol, which can break down skin collagen, the protein that keeps your skin supple and elastic. Sleep loss also slows the production of human growth hormone (HGH), which fuels the natural tissue repair and rejuvenation process that the body would normally be undergoing while you slept. Without it, there's a decrease in muscle mass, your skin gets thinner, and your bones get weaker, thereby accelerating and exacerbating the aging process.

SLEEP AND IMMUNE RESILIENCE

As we've seen in the case of a pandemic—the ultimate test of our immune strength and resilience—sleeping more and better may very well save your life. There's a reason why more and more doctors are recommending sleep as a preventative remedy for widespread viral infection: It's one of the most influential regulators of your immune system.

Your immune system is the original third-shift worker, punching in as you drift off to sleep. It takes advantage of your downtime to repair damaged cells, gain ground in the fight against disease or lingering infection, and manufacture and stockpile protective, infection-fighting molecules, namely cytokine antibodies. Cytokines are kind of like all-purpose modulators in the body, helping you sleep and preparing to protect you from invaders. When you don't get enough sleep, though, your immune system pretty much can't do any of those things. That's why people who don't sleep long or well enough are more likely to get sick, including from viral infections like Covid-19. And when they do get sick, they get sicker and take longer to recover.

In fact, the evidence is so clear that routinely sleeping less than six hours a night compromises your immune system and increases your risk of cancer that the World Health Organization has classified any form of nighttime shiftwork as a probable carcinogen. (The only exception to this is for people with genetic variants on ADRB1 or other genes that allow for less sleep—but this is *not* most of us!)

The biggest problem with dysregulated sleep, or sleep that is out of rhythm, is that it leads to a *dysregulated immune system*. Oftentimes we talk about making your immune system stronger, "boosting" it to fight off whatever comes its way. But another, more accurate way to think of it is having an immune system that knows how to deploy a modulated, measured response, especially in the event of a catastrophic assault such as a novel virus infection. As scientists and doctors discovered when looking at the mortality patterns of Covid-19 (as well as other endemic viruses such as SARS, MERS, and avian flu, in addition to some non-infectious diseases like multiple sclerosis and pancreatitis), a common, often fatal complication they found is called a "cytokine storm." This is when the body launches an *overly* aggressive attack on the virus, unleashing so many cytokines at once that the body sustains too much damage from the resulting inflammation. So while cytokines can be beneficial, particularly when deployed in just the right amount, too many at once can overwhelm the immune system and the body.

When it comes to our immune system, more is not always better. Moderation, modulation, and resilience, however, is. Sleep has the power to equip our body with the best defense system possible.

So while we'll be making a ton of recommendations for building your new sleep-better protocol, which includes fun stuff like building a sleep sanctuary, playing around with sleep-tracking or sleep-aiding gadgets and apps, and trying out natural supplements, we have a bigger, life-saving goal in mind. Don't get us wrong—those remedies can work! But the most powerful, effective thing you can do is to get in rhythm. It's the best medicine that (little to no) money can buy, available to most people, most of the time.

THE CURE-ALL POWER OF RHYTHM

You now know that being out of rhythm steals from your health, moving system by system to compromise things like your heart, brain, circulation, immune response, sexual health, hormones, and weight. But, like an equal and opposite antidote, getting back into rhythm restores and improves these vital functions. It means you'll have the right amount of hormones at the right time of day, which send the correct messages to the right bits of the body. That fires up your metabolism to the appropriate levels at the appropriate moments, which then processes and distributes nutrients effectively and efficiently. That in turn keeps your brain sharp, your heart strong, your skin supple, your immune system resilient, your mood balanced, and your ability to cope with stress—in its many, many forms—even-keeled and hardy.

Best of all, being in sync means that you're getting a nightly dose of good quality, restorative sleep. Scientists may not yet know exactly why we sleep, but they've seen in no uncertain terms that if we are cycling through all the stages of sleep, meaning we're getting deep sleep and enough of it, then we're treated to a whole-body refresh, repair, and reset process every single night. This magical nighttime elixir enhances just about every facet of our health: It boosts our energy levels, helps us lose weight, protects our hearts, strengthens our immunity, rebalances our hormones, improves our ability to focus, clears our minds, raises our spirits, helps us take challenges in stride, keeps us looking and feeling younger, and helps us live longer.

The biggest reason why sleep is so beneficial for your physiology is because it's an opportunity for the cleanup crews to come in and put things back together after the wear and tear of the day. When you get sufficient uninterrupted, deep sleep:

- Your brain creates more **brain-derived neurotrophic factor (BDNF)**. This is a special protein that repairs your brain cells, increases the growth of new brain cells, improves learning and memory, protects you from Alzheimer's disease, and works as a natural antidepressant with the ability to reverse chronic anxiety and depression.
- Your brain has a chance to organize and store all the information it's taken in, which in turn helps you retain new facts, process new memories and integrate them with old ones, and find solutions to problems. Trillions of nerve cells literally rewire themselves to

map out what you've learned,[18] making new connections,
reminding the brain of stored older memories,[19] and clearing out
old or unused information routes (called synapses) to allow for
more efficient brain function the next day.[20]

- You get your daily brain deep-clean care of the glymphatic
  system, a primarily nocturnal, drain-like process that uses
  cerebral spinal fluid to flush waste from your brain, including
  proteins that form Alzheimer's-causing plaque.[21]
- Off-duty brain cells are able to give their employees much-
  needed rest, including mitochondria, the energy-makers of
  your cells, which are key for optimal physiological function.
  These off-duty cells also clear out cellular waste and replenish
  the materials they need to transmit messages throughout the
  body.[22]
- Your gut maintains a better balance of beneficial bacteria,
  specifically in the Verrucomicrobia strain, which is believed to
  be linked to better cognitive function.
- You have better overall gut health, which in turn regulates your
  digestion, immune system, emotional response, and hormonal
  balance.
- Your neurons, or brain cells, break out their repair kits to give
  your DNA a nightly patching up from the damage that simply
  being awake inflicts—and would otherwise accumulate over
  time to unsafe, disease-causing levels.[23]
- Your cardiovascular system resumes a cool, calm baseline,
  leading to a natural drop in blood pressure in those with normal
  or high blood pressure, as well as a slight but beneficial
  reduction in heart rate.[24]
- Your capillaries, arterioles, and arteries—your body's blood,
  oxygen, and nutrient superhighways—have a chance to repair,
  heading off things like heart disease, hypertension, and insulin
  resistance.[25]

- Your immune system reinforces its defenses against infections and chronic inflammation by manufacturing invader-fighting cells, which it can deploy in a modulated fashion.
- Melatonin—the hormone responsible for sleep—slows the multiplication of many types of cancer cells, triggers cancer cell self-destruction (aka apoptosis), and deprives tumors of the blood supply they need to grow.
- Your endocrine system recalibrates your hormones, restoring any previously disrupted levels to normal (especially in the case of testosterone).[26]
- You get an infusion of beneficial hormones that bolster reproductive development, fertility, cell reproduction and regeneration, muscle repair, and bone density.[27]

A PILL ISN'T GOING TO GET YOU THERE

According to a 2018 *Consumer Reports* survey, 80 percent of polled adults admitted to having an issue with sleep at least once a week, and of those people, about one-third of them said that they had at one point that year taken a sleep aid—either over-the-counter (OTC) or prescription—to help.[28] Based on that number, the researchers concluded that as many as 50 million adults in the United States used sleep aids that year. That very large number says a few things to us: (1) Sleep is clearly an enormous and pervasive issue, (2) If you're taking pharmaceutical sleeping aids, you're definitely not alone, and (3) We can do a lot better when it comes to effectively and sustainably addressing issues with sleep. That's because pharmaceutical sleep aids, whether OTC or prescribed by a doctor, are troubling for a number of reasons. These include:

■ **Sleeping Pills Are Not Solving Your Sleep Problem:**
Only about a third of people who said they took sleep medications reported that they got good or excellent sleep on those nights. Six out of ten people reported feeling drowsy, confused, or forgetful the next day. And researchers who reviewed sleep drugs for the most recent treatment guidelines from the American Academy of Sleep Medicine found that some sleep aids only increase your total sleep time by 20 to 30 minutes, while others barely performed better than a placebo.[29] They also noted that most of the commonly used drugs, especially OTC sleeping pills, are not intended to be used long-term and have "shockingly little" published research to even support the efficacy of their short-term use.[30]

It also doesn't take a sleep scientist to deduce that by taking a pill, you're not addressing the root cause of your sleep problems. As we've said before, disrupted sleep is a symptom of something else being off-balance in your body. Merely obliterating that symptom won't get you any closer to better health or better sleep.

- **Sleeping Pills Are Causing You More (Life-Threatening) Problems:** *All* sleep medications come with considerable side effects. These commonly include dizziness, daytime drowsiness, headache, digestive issues, changes in appetite, dry mouth, gas, heartburn, impairment the following day (feeling fuzzy-headed and difficulty focusing, in particular), stomach pain, uncontrollable shaking, weakness, and difficulty breathing. These risks intensify significantly if you combine these medications with other prescription medications, recreational drugs, or alcohol, which one out of ten people have admitted to doing in the name of falling asleep, according to a *Consumer Reports* survey.[31]

The FDA also now requires the makers of many sleeping pills to disclose that these medications can cause parasomnias— that is, sleep behaviors that may cause you to walk, eat, have sex, and even drive while sleeping or semi-asleep. Sleep amnesia, or waking up and not remembering where you are, is another reported side effect. It's not exactly a surprise then that people who take sleeping pills are nearly twice as likely to be in a car crash—just as likely as someone driving with a blood alcohol level over the legal limit.[32] And if you take certain sleeping pills over a period of time, especially benzodiazepines such as Xanax, Valium, Doral, Halcion, ProSom, and Restoril, or sedatives for longer than the typically recommended seven to ten days, your body builds up a tolerance, requiring you to take higher and higher doses in order to get the same effect, which can also cause amplified side effects.

Complicating matters is the fact that it takes some people, especially women and those over age 65, longer to metabolize the active ingredients in these pills, meaning their blood levels remain elevated much longer, leading to a greater risk of impaired driving, falls, and other accidents. And even though the FDA recently issued a new warning about sleeping pills and driving, advising people to take half the dose previously recommended, these medications are not always prescribed or taken as advised.

While the FDA has also recommended smaller doses for people over the age of 65, the side effects of these sleep medications, like an increased risk of excessive drowsiness, unsteadiness, and confusion, make it more likely that people in this vulnerable demographic could fall and suffer broken bones and brain injuries, as well as exacerbate any existing memory problems or cognitive impairment. In a 2017 analysis of people 65 and older, those who were taking sleeping drugs recommended by their doctor over a two-week period were 34 percent more likely to fall than those who weren't.[33] The Mayo Clinic is now phasing out the use of sleep medications such as Ambien because of recent findings that hospital patients who took the drug (under the generic name zolpidem) were four times more likely to experience injury-sustaining falls than those who did not take the drug during their stay.[34]

- **Sleeping Pills Are the New Opioids:** Perhaps the most alarming observation about sleep medications, notably benzodiazepines, is that they share many of the same characteristics as opioids, including their frequency of prescription, highly addictive qualities, and stark mortality rates.[35] Between 1996 and 2013, the number of American adults who filled benzodiazepine prescriptions increased by 67 percent, from 8.1 million to 13.5 million.[36] During that time, there has been an eightfold rise in overdoses.[37] It's also estimated that more than 30 percent of overdoses involving opioids also involve benzodiazepines.[38]

If you are currently taking medication to help with your sleep issues, we recommend working with your health care practitioner to gradually decrease your dose as you introduce new sleep-promoting habits and leave behind those that have been diminishing your sleep. This is not only safer but will also help guard you against "rebound insomnia," a commonly reported phenomenon of sleep issues that get worse than when they originally began after the sudden removal of sleep medication. Additionally, eliminating these medications from your system will further help your body recalibrate and find its natural sleep-inclined rhythm.

DON'T LET SLEEP STRESS YOU OUT:
ORTHOSOMNIA

There's a newly observed phenomenon in the sleep world called "orthosomnia," which describes the obsession to get the "best" sleep, oftentimes causing people to stress out so much about getting to bed that they don't sleep well. It doesn't help that with tracking technology you can now see almost every nuance of your night in bed coupled with an actual "sleep score." While we wanted to give you a little tough love so that you'll get your act together when it comes to getting better rest at night, we don't want that to *interfere* with your sleep. We get that wellness recommendations can bring with them the pressure to do things "perfectly," or the fear of what might happen if you don't. But rest assured (literally!), this book is not about the "best" sleep, namely because there is no such thing. It's merely about getting *better* sleep, because any step toward improved sleep is a step toward improved health. We recognize that real life doesn't always allow for perfection to exist (nor would we want it to), and there's definitely no medal for doing everything "right." There is, however, a reward for doing your best to make a few simple changes to your habits.

Remember: Sleep is a normal biological process that your body wants you to have. Together, we're going to get you back in tune with that rhythm. And once we do, your body will sleep without your having to think about it, plan about it, or stress about it, because that's what a balanced body does. At the end of the day, it's just another night for the books—certainly nothing worth losing sleep over.

CHAPTER 2

GETTING TO KNOW YOUR SLEEP

The fact that you're having trouble with sleep is really just your body telling you that there's something else going on. In traditional Chinese medicine, symptoms are considered guideposts that are pointing to some underlying imbalance. So when Frank meets with a patient, he's looking at sleep as a *clue* of what might be going on, not necessarily as the central issue itself (though, yes, it can be an issue in its own right). That's why when someone presents with not-great sleep, he's looking deeper at whether it could be the result of digestive issues, a hormonal imbalance, or habits that are scrambling proper circadian rhythm.

Luckily, most health-related stumbling blocks present themselves with certain patterns. Because of this, one of Frank's favorite take-home diagnostic tools is a quiz. It allows you to take a deeper look at your ailments and complaints, while illuminating what they have in common. The quiz that follows is to help you more closely examine your own sleep and *why* you're not sleeping. The simple and universal answer is that you're out of sync. But there are a few specific root causes that actively disrupt your daily rhythm and, as a downstream consequence, your sleep. We like to call this finding your Not-Sleeping Type. The types of root causes include:

Stress/Anxiety
Rhythm
Environment
Hormones
Nutrition

Understanding the nature of your particular imbalance (or imbalances—there are often more than one) will help direct you toward the most effective, beneficial habit changes to be found in the following chapters.

WHAT'S YOUR NOT-SLEEPING TYPE?

Go through each section, answer the questions, then tally the number of *yes* responses you have for each. Three or more *yes*es in a section indicate that that root cause is an issue for you. More than one culprit cause may apply to you. If that is the case, don't get overwhelmed. This quiz is not intended to give you a label or make you feel guilt or shame. Rather, it's a tool to give you more specific direction as you track down what's disrupting your sleep. Try to see this insight as empowering instead of limiting. If more than one category does apply to you, take it slow—focus on the root cause for which you scored the highest, then gradually add more habits to address the remaining issues. It will also be particularly helpful for you to go through The Reset (page 225), which is beneficial for all not-sleeping types.

Stress/Anxiety:

1. Do you wake up in the middle of the night and have trouble falling back asleep?

2. Do you have trouble falling asleep or lie in bed wishing you could fall asleep?

3. Do you have difficulty switching off your thoughts before bed?

4. Do you often go to bed angry, anxious, or with unresolved arguments or deadlines?

5. Do you feel nervous, on edge, or anxious during the day?

6. Do you feel restless and as though you can't keep still?

7. Do you clench your teeth at night?

8. Do you often feel like you're not in control?

9. Do you use alcohol or nicotine to help you cope with uncomfortable feelings? What about THC or CBD? (The latter two can actually be good sleep aids, which we'll discuss more on page 158, but we also want to get to the root of your not-sleeping issue.)

10. Do you often feel afraid that something terrible may happen?

Score: _____

Rhythm:

1. Do your bedtime and/or wake times vary from day to day?

2. Do your mealtimes vary from day to day?

3. Do you eat a meal or snacks within two hours of going to bed?

4. Do you try to "catch up" on sleep on the weekends?

5. Do you often use electronics like a television, computer, or smartphone within two hours of going to sleep?

6. Do you expose yourself to bright light in the middle of the night (looking at your phone, turning on the light to go to the bathroom)?

7. Are there still sources of artificial light in your bedroom even after you've turned out the light?

8. Do you rigorously exercise in the evening?
9. Do hours pass before you're exposed to natural light in the morning?
10. Do you spend a majority of your day under artificial light?

Score: _____

Environmental:

1. Are there sources of artificial light in your bedroom after you've turned out the light?
2. Do you have multiple electronics plugged in in your bedroom?
3. Are there outside noises that you feel like you have to "tune out" at night (garbage trucks, neighbors, appliances running)?
4. Does your bedroom tend to be warm?
5. Do you sleep with the windows closed year-round?
6. Do you wake up with a sore back or neck?
7. Do you wake up sweating at night from overly warm bedding?
8. Do you or your partner snore?
9. Do you sleep with a partner who is on a different sleep schedule from you?
10. Do you have a pet who sleeps in your bed?

Score: _____

Nutritional:

1. Is dinner typically your largest and heaviest meal of the day?
2. Do you eat foods made with sugar?
3. Do you drink caffeine after noon, or eat caffeine-containing foods such as chocolate, coffee-flavored desserts, or soda?
4. Do you drink alcohol more than three times a week or smoke tobacco?

5. Do you tend to eat spicy foods at night?
6. Do you experience reflux or heartburn after eating?
7. Do you frequently experience gas and bloating soon after you eat?
8. Do you frequently feel tired or get brain fog after eating?
9. Do you have constipation or loose stools?
10. Do you take general medications, supplements, or recreational drugs that could disrupt your sleep?

Score: _____

Hormonal:

1. Are you in menopause, perimenopause, or andropause?
2. Have you been diagnosed with PCOS?
3. Are your periods irregular?
4. Do you experience PMS?
5. Do you have problems sleeping during the week or so before your period?
6. Are you gaining weight around your midsection?
7. Do you frequently feel irritable, anxious, or depressed?
8. Do you have low libido?
9. Do you often feel fatigued?
10. Do you often experience brain fog?

Score: _____

INSOMNIACS WELCOME HERE

If you struggle with insomnia, or the inability to fall asleep and/or stay asleep multiple nights a week, you're probably thinking that this is your not-sleeping type. Nope! Not to make you feel too normal and optimistic, but if you experience either ongoing (chronic) or temporary (acute) bouts of insomnia, you're no different than anyone else with less-than-ideal quality of sleep. You're just struggling with a symptom of being out of rhythm. And like any symptom, you have to treat the root cause—which is most likely one of the aforementioned not-sleeping issues. Luckily, this can most likely be done using the protocol you create from this book.

When going through the new habits in the next four chapters, we recommend focusing on those that help quell anxiety, shift your beliefs and attitudes about sleep, create a consistent sleep schedule, and get sufficient movement during the day. We also highly recommend downloading a CBT-I app. CBT-I is cognitive-behavioral therapy specifically for insomnia, which is recommended as the first line of treatment and can be very effective. The therapy helps you identify thoughts and behaviors that can worsen your sleep issues, and then replaces them with habits that promote better sleep. (Sound familiar?) Apps such as Sleepio or CBT-I Coach can be a nice supplement to the sleep-better protocol that you build here. Of course, if you continue to struggle with insomnia—or rather the issues that underlie it, such as anxiety—then we encourage you to seek out a professional who can help.

TRACKING YOUR PROGRESS
WITH SLEEP TECH

We're big fans of tracking your sleep, whether you're using a device, an app on your phone, or a good old-fashioned sleep journal. That's because the more information you have about your sleep, the better insight you'll have about whether your sleep protocol is working, or if you need to make any adjustments. You also get real-time feedback about the effect certain things have on your sleep, such as that glass of wine (probably negative) or that bonus stretching session you snuck in before bed (probably positive). Ultimately, sleep tracking is one of the best tools around when it comes to personalizing and optimizing your sleep wellness.

Choosing a Sleep-Tracking Method

Sleep trackers each have different mechanisms for gauging these things: Some devices have a sensor that rests on your pulse and uses your heart rate variability (HRV) for extrapolating when you fall asleep and what stage of sleep you're in. Others monitor your breathing rate (also using HRV as a gauge), while more simple technology, such as apps, rely on motion or sound sensing. These technologies run the gamut from costing a few hundred dollars to being completely free and, as you may imagine, range in terms of accuracy and the detail of their feedback.

Here's a breakdown of some of the sleep trackers that are currently on offer:

- Physical trackers
  - Oura ring (tracks sleep + HRV through a ring worn on the finger)

- Whoop band (tracks sleep + HRV through a wrist strap)
- Fitbit bands
- Garmin watches (e.g., Forerunner 945)
- Apple Watch (caveat: It has to be charged every day or every other day, so wearing it at night can be cumbersome)
- Under-mattress sensors (don't require you to wear anything, but sometimes can get confused by a user's partner or pets)
  - Emfit
  - Beddit
  - Withings
- Fully app-based
  - SleepCycle
  - Pillow
  - Sleep Score
- Old-school analog
  - Use the template we've provided for The Reset (page 227) to use a pen-and-paper approach.

As for choosing one, it really comes down to personal preference. Remember, there's no winning sleep, you can't buy your way to better sleep, and no sleep tracker is going to make you put down the cookie and pick up the yoga mat. It comes down to what will empower you to make the changes you need to make. It's worth pointing out that none of these technologies is considered the gold standard when it comes to getting the most reliable, accurate data. That would be a polysomnogram (PSG), which you would get in a sleep lab in order to detect a clinical sleep disorder, such as sleep apnea. However, what you can start to monitor—and what is just as actionable and useful as anything you'd learn from a lab (if not more so because you're combining this info with new, powerful habits)—are *patterns*. Ideally, you want to see a pattern of improvement. You want to watch how your sleep changes from night to night in response to changing certain variables in your life. This means comparing data to itself with week-over-week improvements or looking at specific days when you drink alcohol versus don't drink alcohol or when you stop coffee early versus drinking later in the evening to understand how that habit is affecting you.

The best tracking system for you is the one that you'll use consistently and gives you the kind of feedback that motivates you to make good, sleep-promoting decisions throughout the day.

DON'T LET TRACKING TRIP YOU UP

If you're the type of person who will get obsessive about your results or will shame spiral after a less-than-great night of sleep, then give yourself permission to step away from the tracker. This feedback should help you measure success and feel good when you see the needle move, not prompt you to get mired in how little REM sleep you got one night and how it's all your fault because of what you ate for lunch. Ideally, you can look at your data in a non-judgmental, even compassionate way, just observing where things are and knowing that they can only get better from here. But if you're having a tough time getting into that headspace, then tracking may not be for you. In that case, stay the course with your sleep protocol and go by how you feel: Better rested? Better digestion? Better focus? Take the shame out of the game and focus on how you can start feeling better.

Neil is a great example of this—he has an admittedly complicated relationship with sleep trackers because he tends to obsess over metrics...then get sick of them and give up. The solution that works for him is using a sleep a tracker every few months for a few weeks to reset, especially when he has a hunch that something is off (he's getting sick more often, has a harder time waking up, etc.). Combined with examining his habits (like whether going back to drinking full-strength coffee is having a detrimental effect), he can start to get an idea of how his sleep is falling short, especially if it's slipping consistently in his bed and wake times, or lack of restful sleep in between.

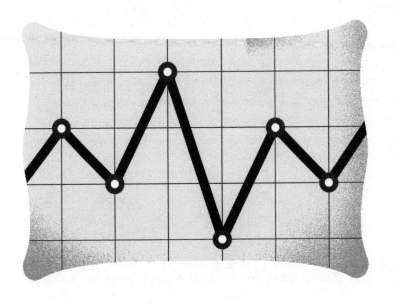

DECODING YOUR SLEEP

Just like you can track your heart rate and calories burned during exercise, route a run while also calculating your biometrics, or log your meals and macronutrients, new sleep technology and apps allow you to get an even clearer picture of what's happening after you drift off to sleep. For the most part, sleep-tracking technologies—especially those with sensor capabilities—are registering your **sleep latency,** or the amount of time it takes you to fall asleep; the **stages of sleep,** or the length of time you spend in each phase of sleep, such as deep sleep and REM; **total sleep,** or the duration of time you're asleep; and **restfulness,** which measures how frequently you wake in the night.

This data isn't 100 percent scientifically ironclad, but it does lend insight into what's going on with your sleep. Here's how to make sense of the numbers so you can gauge where you are on the road to good rest:

- **Sleep latency:** A healthy, in-rhythm body can shut down and effortlessly drift to sleep between **5 and 30 minutes** after lying down in bed, with 30 being acceptable and 5 to 15 being optimal. If it takes you longer, refer back to "What's Your Not-Sleeping Type" on page 45.
- **The stages of sleep:** Your sleep at night is a rhythm within a rhythm. As you rest, **you cycle through four stages of sleep, ideally four or five times each night**. Because the body accomplishes different tasks during each stage, it's essential to your health as well as your overall rhythm that each of these stages is not only reached but also as uninterrupted as possible. These stages include
  - **Stage 1 (NREM):** This is when you transition between wakefulness and sleep. Your breathing and heart rate slow, your muscles begin to relax, and your core temperature dips.

At this point you can still easily be woken by distractions and noise.

- **Stage 2 (NREM):** You are still in light sleep but now your brain waves slow down and your body enters a deep state of relaxation. Your brain activity is dominated by theta waves, which foster learning, memory, and intuition. During this stage, theta waves are interrupted by short bursts of waves called spindles, which are believed to aid the consolidation of information and memories.

- **Stage 3 (NREM):** This is the beginning of deep sleep, also known as slow-wave or delta sleep. Brain waves slow further; your heart rate and respiration slow dramatically; your body temperature cools further; and your muscles are completely relaxed. This is when human growth hormone is released (essential for keeping the body supple and resilient) and the regenerative processes happen. The brain begins to "detoxify" using the glymphatic system (waste removal for the central nervous system) and DNA repair is at its peak. Surges of energy have also been detected during this time, as the body seems to store energy for the next day.

- **Stage 4 (REM):** This is when the brain almost exclusively produces slow, impactful delta waves, which are generated in deepest meditation and dreamless sleep. They are to credit for sleep feeling restorative and for us waking up feeling refreshed. While the rest of your muscles are temporarily paralyzed (besides your respiratory and cardiovascular functions), vivid dreaming hits its stride and your brain waves look similar to those when you're awake. This stage is named for the "rapid eye movements" that occur while a person is experiencing REM sleep. The REM portion of your sleep cycle lengthens as the night progresses, allowing your brain to perform the maintenance that benefits your learning, memory, and mood. Interruptions during this part of sleep—as a result of your snoring, your partner's snoring, sudden noises, anxious awakenings, muscle spasms—deprive the brain from sorting through daily events and making cognitive connections, ultimately leading to a range of consequences from difficulty focusing and learning to depression.

Hitting all four stages of sleep is where quantity of sleep and quality meet. In order to hit the deepest, most restful sleep, your body has to pass through all the other stages first. The order goes: 1, 2, 3, 1, 3, 2, 1, REM. No matter what you do, you can't rush this process, and you can't cheat sleep.

Ideally, you would spend one to two hours in deep sleep for every seven to nine hours of one night's rest.

- **Total sleep:** Pretty straightforward: Total sleep simply refers to how much sleep, including all the stages, that you get a night.

HOW MUCH TOTAL SLEEP DO I REALLY NEED?

Even as two people who are in the business of helping people sleep better, we can honestly say that we don't really know yet how much or how little sleep we need. So for now, we're sticking with what The National Sleep Foundation recommends, which is **seven to nine hours of sleep per night for adults**. We like that range because we know that dipping down to six hours is enough to trigger all the side effects of sleep deprivation (see page 15), and that overdoing it with more than nine hours is correlated to an increased risk of cardiovascular disease and death. Not to worry, though, this does not apply to little kids and teenagers, whom we'll address in Chapter 8. And no, you do not get a free sleep-less pass if you're over the age of 65, which we'll also address in that chapter. Though, if you are an

---

athlete or frequently exercise at a high intensity and are putting your body under significant physiological stress, you may need more sleep to aid in recovery.

But, as Neil can attest as someone who has been in your position, it can be helpful to initially focus less on a magic number and more on *more and better sleep* than what you're currently getting.

■ **Restfulness:** Many sleep-tracking apps and devices will show you when in the night you wake up prematurely. As you well know by now, disrupting the sleep stages can be more than just getting up to pee/check your phone/double-check your to-do list. It can also interrupt the series of events that add up to your sleep rhythm and all the essential physiological benefits that come with it. Waking from time to time and immediately drifting back to sleep is a normal part of adult slumber. In fact, most adults wake a few times a night as we transition from one sleep cycle to the next every 90 minutes or so. However, if your wakefulness is a result of physical discomfort, a noisy partner, your own snoring/sleep apnea, too much light in the room, your bed being too hot, or mental noise (all common reasons for middle-of-the-night waking), then make sure that your sleep protocol addresses these issues (because we have solutions!).

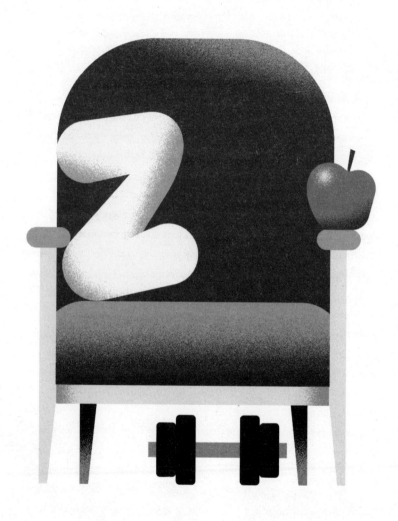

CHAPTER 3

RESETTING THE CLOCK
WITH NEW HABITS

No matter how out of rhythm you are, **your Master Clock can reset itself.** And *you* have the power to make that happen—without prescription medications, extensive therapy, or expensive technology. You have the ability to achieve easy, effortless, satisfying sleep—the way nature intended it to be. The solution? New and simple daily habits.

Your primary day-night rhythm is affected by pretty much everything you do, day *and* night—the foods you eat, the behaviors you engage in, and the environment you surround yourself with. By curating a new roster of sleep-promoting habits in these categories, you'll be actively bringing yourself back to where your body needs to be in order to get a good night's rest. Think of it this way: Every day, you have 24 hours' worth of opportunities to shift that rhythm back into place.

Over the next four chapters, you are going to build your own sleep-better protocol. To do that, you're going to take your knowledge of (1) your not-sleeping type, (2) your unique physiological needs when it comes to sleep (regardless of whether you're a night owl or morning lark—more on this on page 71), and (3) your own personal preferences and lifestyle inclinations (because we're realists, and we've seen what's happened to all of your New Year's resolutions . . .).

Then *you* will be the one choosing what to add and what to take away.

All of the shifts we recommend are designed to remove any obstructions that are keeping you from sleep, while also nourishing you where you might be deficient. Over time, they are meant to keep your Master Clock entrained to the proper day-night rhythm, your systems in comfortable homeostasis, your hormones balanced, and your nervous system in check, while helping you to feel less anxious and stressed and more cool and calm.

The most important thing you have to do is commit. This may be a simple process, but it's not just a quick fix. It involves making some profound, perhaps even uncomfortable changes, but the benefits are abundant.

Just remember:

The discomfort will be temporary.
The results will be almost immediate.
The consequences will be powerful and long-term.
You get to call the shots.
And if you trip up, you can always get started again.

If you take the suggestions in the following chapters one day at a time, you will soon be able to hear your own rhythm and the beat that your body and mind need to feel healthy and strong again.

BUILDING YOUR SLEEP-BETTER PROTOCOL

Over the next four chapters, we've laid out some of the most impactful habit shifts you can make to finally get better sleep. They fall into the following four categories, which reflect the main factors that affect your primary rhythm:

LIVE TO SLEEP
MOVE TO SLEEP
EAT TO SLEEP
SANCTUARY TO SLEEP

Think of the following as your à la carte sleep menu: Take a look. See what sounds good. Ask yourself: *What could be getting in the way of my sleep that needs to be removed? And what might be missing that needs to be added?* Then mix and match, because none of these recommendations can hurt, and all of them will help you sleep better than you are now. You just have to commit.

You can start small with a few new habits and layer in additional ones over time, or you can dive into the deep end with a whole new slate of shifts that target the most significant sleep-affecting areas of your life. That's up to you, how much of a change you need, and how quickly you need it. Either way, we highly recommend getting a jump start with The Reset (page 225) to build the strongest rhythm-correcting foundation possible and see satisfying results almost immediately.

Ideally, your protocol will have two levels.

Level 1: Universal Basics

These are the recommendations that benefit everyone—things like making sure your bedroom is dark, your mattress is supportive, and you're not on your phone up until the moment you go to bed. But while these steps will help and are important pieces of your sleep hygiene, they won't necessarily be the entire solution if you're also struggling with underlying hormone- or microbiome-related issues.

Level 2: Personalized Prescription

These are the recommendations that are tailored to your specific not-sleeping type, while also delivering a more powerful, targeted punch. They are the steps that will help completely reset and recalibrate your biological systems so that they're once again in rhythm and ready to support sleep.

Here are the plans for each type:

Stress/Anxiety: Calm down sympathetic nervous system and decrease cortisol at night

Rhythm: Synchronize with the sun, institute a consistent sleep schedule, and establish a daily eating rhythm

Environment: Remove obstacles and change other factors in the immediate sleep environment (bedroom) that inhibit sleep

Hormones: Strengthen natural hormonal rhythm and add habits that encourage balanced hormone production

Nutrition: Correct microbiome imbalances and avoid foods that negatively affect sleep

A few more things to keep in mind when building your protocol:

We're not purists: These recommendations are meant for real life. Yes, we like certain sleep apps, such as those that encourage a deeper level of sleep with soundwaves or provide guided meditations. We also suggest not keeping your phone next to your bed as you sleep because of things like melatonin-disrupting blue light and EMFs, short for electromagnetic fields. We're not trying to be annoying. We're just recognizing that in the pursuit of sleep, there is no such thing as the "perfect" choices, just the perfect choices for you. If you're digging yourself out of a pretty big sleep deficit, those apps might be more beneficial than going into total monk mode immediately out of the gate. Choose new habits that feel good and help you sleep—if they work, then don't sweat the small stuff.

Once again, this is real life: We'll say it again: The only way you can effect change in your sleep is to create change in your life—your very busy, very unpredictable, very real life. By committing to these habits as consistently as you possibly can and for as long as you can, you'll be setting yourself up for success when the unexpected inevitably comes down the road. These habits are meant to work together to create a new-normal baseline for your rhythms. That way, when the occasional late night out/kid throwing up all night/studying bender does come up, it won't create as much chaos. And you'll have the tools to get yourself back on track (and maybe even buy yourself a little more security, if you're able to plan in advance). Bottom line: Life happens, hiccups will happen, and these habits will help you be better prepared.

ABC (Always Be Considering) sleep: Managing sleep is an all-day process; the choices you make throughout your 24-hour circadian cycle affect how you sleep at night. That's why the habits you'll be choosing from are meant to be incorporated at different times of the day in order to be in sync with your rhythm and give you a day and night's worth of continuous sleep support. To help you figure out when these habits are most effectively applied, we've included the following icons for each of the entries:

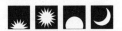

Don't skimp on your goal: While we want you to focus on getting **more and better** sleep than you were previously getting, ideally you should keep working toward getting **seven to nine hours of sleep per night.** It may not happen right away, but that's the ideal.

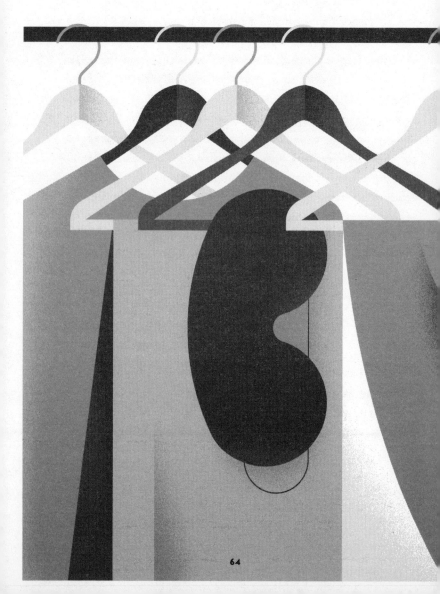

CHAPTER 4

LIVE TO SLEEP

The secret to achieving the most refreshing, revitalizing, reinvigorating, all-night-long, up-with-the-birds sleep possible is simple but powerful: You have to live to sleep. You have to align the behaviors and practices that you engage in throughout the day with getting superior sleep results at night. Because how you move, act, and feel throughout the day sets the stage for how well your body is able to receive sleep.

The habits in this chapter are meant to be reached for throughout the day and have the cumulative benefit of re-syncing your sleep cycle and keeping it there. And they have as much to do with *what* you're doing as *when* you're doing it so that your Master Clock begins to find its more natural groove.

Also, know that these habits come with unavoidable (positive) side effects: If you experience less anxiety, more calm, increased energy, decreased stress, more frequent orgasms, and the ability to breathe more deeply, please call your doctor—and tell them it may be a while until you see them next.

CHANGE YOUR MIND ABOUT SLEEP

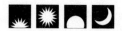

In this chapter—and the chapters that follow—we present some majorly powerful, scientifically proven, expert-endorsed, life-changing behavioral shifts that you can make in your life to positively affect your sleep. But the most important habit you could possibly adopt in order to ensure your success is not physical; it's mental. If you're not 100 percent mentally committed to making these changes, then they're not going to be very effective. That's why the first habit we suggest adding to your protocol is *changing your attitudes and beliefs about sleep.*

If you have been telling yourself these self-defeating (and false) stories about sleep, then it's time to let them go:

- I have no control over my sleep.
- My mother/father had this problem, and that's why I have this problem.
- It's just normal as you get older. (Something we'll dig even deeper into in Chapter 8.)
- It's not that important.
- It's not connected to the rest of my health.
- I'll just catch up on sleep on the weekend.
- I need sleep medication in order to solve the problem.
- I need to rely on a sleep specialist and their recommendations, not my own tools.
- I am my label: insomniac/frequent waker/light sleeper, etc.

Now, use some positive affirmations about sleep. Repeat after us:

- Sleep is affecting every aspect of my health.
- I have the power to improve my sleep.
- I have the tools to improve my sleep.
- Everything I do throughout the day affects my sleep, for better or worse.

One way to keep yourself feeling optimistic as you navigate this new path is to think about your improvement as you would the numbers on a scale. Your weight is not designed to be the be all and end-all indicator of health. But it does allow you to see progress. Getting an extra 15 minutes of sleep is a small percentage of your entire night's rest—about as little as 3 percent if you're sleeping eight hours. It's hard to see an extra 3 percent difference in anything in your health: 3 percent better circulation? Three percent better metabolism? But if you saw a 3 percent decrease on the scale, you'd notice it. (It's the equivalent of losing six pounds if you weighed 200.) So that 15 or 30 minutes of quality sleep that you added as part of your commitment to resetting your sleep rhythm is a big relative improvement. And when you compound that over time, the benefits are huge.

END SOCIAL JET LAG TURBULENCE

Our Master Clock thrives on consistency. After all, there's not a lot of variation in when the sun sets and rises. And the sun definitely isn't setting its schedule back a few hours because it wants to go out for a few drinks. We, on the other hand, are more than happy to rearrange our schedules to accommodate our social lives and personal needs. As a result, our sleep-wake schedules are all over the place—later on some nights for dinner plans, studying, or TV binges; earlier some mornings for yoga, school, or meetings; and then a free-for-all on the weekends as we try to make up for the weekday sleep deficit. As a result, we experience what researchers call "social jet lag," or the body-wide chaos that ensues when our social rhythm doesn't match up with our biological one.

The consequences are similar to the jet lag we experience when we travel—fatigue, brain fog, digestive issues, general discombobulation. Now imagine that happening every day, with the effects becoming chronic and more pronounced. A new study has found that an inconsistent sleep schedule coupled with getting different amounts of sleep each night can put you at a higher risk for obesity, high cholesterol, hypertension, high blood sugar, and other metabolic disorders. Another study found that weekday sleep deprivation followed by weekend makeup sleeping may be worse for blood sugar control than just chronic sleep deprivation alone.[39]

Frank has noticed that when many of his patients are experiencing issues with sleep—and the downstream health effects—social jet lag is often to blame. Having a practice in New York City, where schedules and productivity take precedence over observing a consistent, good-for-you rhythm, Frank has a front-row seat to what can happen when social jet lag sets in. And it's not pretty. So let's officially let go of the idea that you can "bank" more sleep on the weekend or make up for what you didn't get during the week. The brain doesn't have a concept of sleep debt that you can pay off in installments.

Then, recognize that one of the most powerful things you can do to get your body back into rhythm is to observe consistent bed- and wake-times. This is also called "sleep stability," and it's one of the cornerstones of cognitive-behavioral therapy for insomniacs. Essentially, it just means choosing a time to go to bed and wake up, then sticking with it every day, including on the weekends.★ The result is getting into a groove that your body understands and anticipates.

★We're not monsters, and thankfully, neither are the researchers who found that giving yourself one lazy morning a week is typically not enough to upset your sleep rhythm. Some people can even bump this up to two, but if sleeping in starts pushing your bedtime later, then come back to your baseline sleep schedule.

CHOOSING THE RIGHT SLEEP SCHEDULE FOR YOU

At the most basic level, there is no complicated formula: Figure out what time you'd like to be up in the morning and work backwards to arrive at your best bedtime, adding in how much sleep you'd ideally get (seven to nine hours) and taking into account that it would ideally be two to three hours after dinnertime. The specific times you choose to go to sleep and wake up are less important than the rhythm and consistency of those things happening.

The other factor to take into account is your chronotype, as in — are you someone who benefits from early rising (a Lark), or is the late night when you thrive (an Owl)? Figuring out your chronotype (page 71) will help give you more insight into how to create a rhythm that works best for your unique physiological preferences.

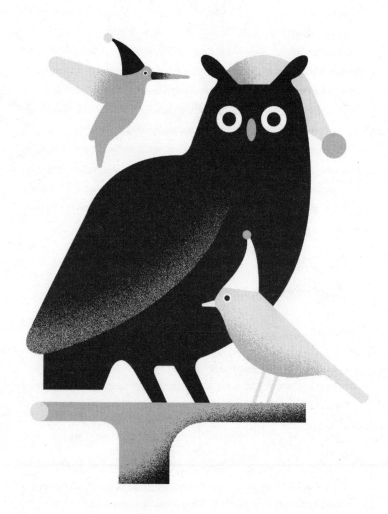

EMBRACE YOUR CHRONOTYPE

Even though we all have an innate 24-hour rhythm, not all of our rhythms are the same. The clearest example of this is the fact that some of us identify as early risers who feel their best when getting up with the sun, while others peak in the deeper hours of the evening. Whether you're in the first group, the second group, or somewhere in between depends on your "chronotype," or your genetically programmed preferences for sleeping and waking during a 24-hour period. Choosing a sleep-wake schedule that takes your chronotype into account will help you arrive at a rhythm that supports when you're naturally inclined to sleep, wake up, and perform.

- **You're a Lark If . . .** (about 20 percent of people)
  - You're up at the crack of dawn, raring to go.
  - You get up before 6 a.m. (without an alarm clock) and tend to get drowsy early in the evening, around 9 p.m.
  - You aren't overly reliant on caffeine in the morning.
  - You are most alert and feel most productive at work a few hours before lunch.
  - You lose your mental sharpness in the afternoon.
- **You're an Owl If . . .** (about 20 percent of people)
  - You enjoy staying up way past midnight.
  - You wake up naturally closer to 10 a.m. and don't want to go to bed before 3 a.m.
  - You need an alarm clock to get you up earlier in the morning and need lots of caffeine to stay alert during the day.

- Your day really only starts to get going in the afternoon—you are alert later in the day and do your most productive work later in the evening.
- **You Could Also Be a Hummingbird** (about 60 percent of people)

While Larks and Owls have set preferences, Hummingbirds fall somewhere in the middle with no strong predilections for what time of day they engage in various activities. Some Hummingbirds are more Lark-ish, and others more Owl-ish.

Can You Hack Your Chronotype?

We get it—there's a distinct advantage to being a Lark. Because of how our society is set up, namely early start times for work and school, Larks tend to get better sleep, and by extension, be healthier and less prone to conditions like heart disease and diabetes. It's hard to be an Owl in a Lark's world. But even though your chronotype is built into your genes, it's technically adjustable. In fact, chronotypes change for all sorts of reasons—the seasons, age, latitude, consistent exposure to bright light at night, and shifting attitudes (commonly the teenage creed: early bedtimes are for little kids). But it's not always for the better—after all, it's a piece of your unique physiology. That's why we recommend first assessing your DNA-determined chronotype and perhaps finding a way to embrace that natural rhythm. However, if it better suits your lifestyle, you can adjust your chronotype—something we're in favor of *if it ultimately means you'll get more sleep.* Just be sure you're being consistent and committing to this new schedule long-term. Otherwise, you risk self-inflicting social jet lag (page 68) and sending your sleep rhythm into a tailspin.

Tips for Shifting Your Chronotype

If You're a Lark:

Spend time outside in the late afternoon or evening. Going for a walk is ideal.

Exercise or increase your activity in the later afternoon or evening.

Socialize in the evenings as a way to naturally energize yourself later in the day.

If You're an Owl:

Dim the lights in your home in the evening.

Sleep with the curtains open so daylight wakes you up, or be sure to expose yourself to early morning light first thing upon waking.

Go for a walk outside as soon as possible after you get up.

Avoid sleeping in on weekends. (Which we know you'll cut back on after addressing social jet lag.)

Don't exercise or engage in stimulating activities like watching television or even doing work in the evening.

If You're a Hummingbird:

Identify whether it would be beneficial for you to shift more toward a Lark or an Owl and follow those corresponding suggestions.

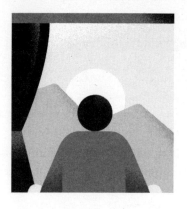

SYNC WITH THE SUN

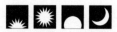

While light is not the only factor that influences your daily rhythms, it is the most important. It's the strongest cue that your body uses to set its clock: If the light is on, it's day; if the light is off, it's night. The only problem is, because of artificial lighting (in your office, on the street, in your bedroom, on your screens), your body can get very mixed messages about what's what. And as you're aware by now, when your day-night rhythm is off, you're going to have trouble falling asleep at night and difficulty getting out of bed in the morning, your cells and systems will no longer be working together as a team, and your overall health will be affected. In fact, this disjointed relationship with day and night is one of the most common root causes of Frank's patients' health issues.

Deeply ingrained in your cells is programming meant to align with the *sun*. The light-sensor cells in your eyes that report their findings to your brain don't know how to distinguish whether light is natural or man-made. As a result, your body gets confused.

- At night: Your body responds to bright light exposure the same way it responds to daylight—suppressing melatonin and doing away with sleep.
- During the day: Your body doesn't know what to do with the not-as-strong-as-the-sun indoor light, leading to less wake-promoting neurotransmitters, and also less serotonin, which not only makes you feel good but is also a precursor to the melatonin your body relies on at night.

Artificial Light, Artificial Rhythm

While miraculous and helpful, our modern light environment—filled with the glare of indoor lights, computer screens, and other devices—has messed with our daily rhythm. With fewer cues from the sun because we're inside most of the day, our brains get confused about when it should be producing melatonin and downcycling for the day. The same goes for when we're sitting in our well-lit homes at night, scrolling through our newsfeed, or watching television. As a result, we're unintentionally manipulating our biological clocks, leaving our bodies with no clue about when it's time to go to sleep.

A recent study illustrates what happens when we introduce artificial light into our daily rhythm: Participants living in a natural environment with more sunlight during the day and essentially no light at night developed a melatonin cycle that began gradually at dusk, peaked around midnight, and ebbed at dawn. But back in the real world, their biological clocks shifted back by two hours, with melatonin only beginning to increase after dark and subside after they woke up in the morning, which is enough to upset even a night owl's rhythm.[40]

In order to correct this, consider going Paleo and take a cue from what our cavemen and cavewomen ancestors would have done. They'd sync with the sun, getting natural light throughout the day and natural darkness in the evening.

We recognize that it's not realistic for you to avoid artificial light completely. But being mindful of your exposure both during the day and at night—along with getting plenty of natural sunlight and darkness—will help re-entrain your rhythm to where nature meant it to be. We'll show you exactly how to do this in "Rise and Shine," below and "Dim with the Dark," page 78.

RISE AND SHINE

Getting a hit of sunshine is nature's way of revving up your entire body into awake-mode and locking it into a 24-hour schedule that delivers more refreshed, energized mornings thanks to better sleep at night. Studies agree that the more exposure to natural sun you get in the morning, the more alert you'll be,[41] and the less stressed and depressed you'll feel.[42] This is owing to a healthy boost of cortisol, plus feel-good hormones serotonin and dopamine and immune-strengthening vitamin D. Basking in the rays during the day is also thought to have a protective effect against artificial light in the evening. That's because when your body establishes a daytime baseline of truly bright light from the sun, the dimmer glow of light bulbs and screens won't have the same disruptively stimulating effect. (Though, that's not a free pass to ignore our advice in the next section, "Dim with the Dark.")

Sleep-Better Solution: Get Some Sun

Within an hour of waking, try to expose yourself to natural light. Open your drapes or curtains to flood your bedroom with sun (as best you can), or better yet, get outside for 30 to 45 minutes. You could even pair this with a morning workout to get an extra boost of energy that's in line with your body's preferred rhythm. Don't worry, even if it's overcast, you'll still get the benefits of morning light because the sun's rays can filter through clouds.

Then throughout the day, re-up your exposure to sunlight as best you can. The ideal is a cumulative two hours' worth of natural sunlight each day, even if it's just sitting by a window or taking a quick walk around the block. This might seem like a chore, but remember that if you work indoors all day, your body isn't getting the correct cues about what it needs to be doing and when. Coordinating check-ins with the sun will ensure that you preserve the rhythm that you're trying so hard to achieve.

LIGHT TIME AT THE RIGHT TIME

One of the most common sleep-related issues that Neil wanted to tackle at Casper was artificial light exposure. He wanted to introduce artificial light in people's environments in a less problematic — and at times, even beneficial — way. He and his team realized that if there was a light that could be programmed to gradually illuminate in the morning instead of an alarm, then your body would naturally transition out of rest and keep its rhythm on track. (They also took it a step further and created the capability for the blue light-free lamp to gradually dim in the evening — more on blue light and its effects on page 78.) These lamps aren't a replacement for natural light, but they're particularly great if you sleep in a dark bedroom. Products we like include:

Totobay Sunrise alarm clock
Casper Glow
Philips Wake-Up light

DIM WITH THE DARK

We once heard it described that light is like a cup of coffee—not necessarily good or bad in and of itself, it just depends on when you have it. And like coffee, natural light can give you a similar rocket fuel-like energetic boost in the morning, a result of its melatonin-suppressing, anti-drowsy effects. But if you get that same dose of artificial light in the evening, your brain becomes wired when it should be winding down for bed, similar to what might happen after a poorly timed latte. As a result, your sleep cycle is pushed later into the evening instead of being synced with the setting of the sun; your body thinks it needs to be asleep for less time than it actually does; and your sleep quality takes a hit.

Here's what to know:

- The connection between too-bright nighttime lighting, sleep disorders, and health risks is so strong that the American Medical Association issued a statement saying as much and calling for the development of alternative lighting technologies that don't interfere with the sleep-wake cycle.
- Any kind of light can suppress melatonin production, but blue light at night is the biggest offender. Blue light refers to the blue wavelengths of light that come from things like electronics with screens and some energy-efficient lighting. Blue light in and of itself isn't bad (the sun is a major source of blue light) but it goes back to the coffee analogy—you don't want its stimulating effects at night.
- Even dim light can get in the way of your circadian rhythm and melatonin production. Researchers have found measures of light as small as 8 lux (about the same as a table lamp) can have an effect on your rhythm. So while things like night-mode settings and blue-light blockers can be beneficial, brightness matters too.

Here's what to do:

- Increase the warm light "night mode" setting on your smartphone, if it has one. (There are plenty of tutorials online for how to do that.)
- Switch to "dark mode" or "night mode" on your desktop, laptop, and other electronics (though this won't address blue light, just the overall brightness).
- Use blue-light filters on your television, smartphone, ebook reader, and other screens (usually just a thin overlay that sits on top of your screen). You could also wear a pair of blue-light-blocking glasses, which are surprisingly reasonable-looking, if not downright cool.
- Avoid screens and bright artificial lights two to three hours before bed. The best way to keep yourself accountable? Set an "electric sundown" alarm, which can either be automatic (some phones can be programmed to switch to dimmer, warmer light after a certain time) or simply an alarm you set for yourself to start dimming the lights.
- Get more natural sunlight exposure throughout the day, which tempers how your body perceives the brightness of artificial light.
- Use more intelligent lighting, such as smart bulbs, which switch between warm, reddish light in the evening and cool, blue-hued tones during the day. They can also be programmed to progressively brighten in the morning and dim in the evening. Some of these lights can connect to apps, through which you can program your home's lighting. Amazon's Alexa and Google's Home Hub both offer this option.

STOP STRESSING ABOUT STRESS

If we had to pick one of the worst offenders to sleep—and there are many—stress would definitely be up there in the power rankings. As Neil can attest personally, and as Frank sees in his practice pretty much every day, stress clearly impacts sleep quality and duration. And at times, it creates a vicious cycle: Stressing out about how stress is causing you to sleep less, in turn, only creates more stress. It's a classic sequence that leaves us "wired and tired." More studies than we can count have confirmed the detrimental connection between stress and sleep, which affects people of all ages, including children, adolescents, and teens struggling with school- and social life-related pressures.

We're guessing that if you've picked up this book, then you don't need a scientist to tell you about the mind-racing, heart-palpitating, chest-tightening grip that stress has on sleep. (Stress/Anxiety is also most likely one of your not-sleeping types.) You're not alone. According to the American Psychological Association, 43 percent of Americans say stress has caused them to lie awake at night at least once a month.

But look—you're never going to completely avoid stress. We are hardwired to experience it in the name of survival. So stressing *less* isn't the solution. Learning to cope with stress, on the other hand, is.

What Is Stress?

In a nutshell: When your brain perceives a "threat," it triggers a cascading chemical reaction that prepares your body to meet that threat. Your adrenal glands pump epinephrine (adrenaline) into your bloodstream, causing your sympathetic nervous system to go into high alert. Your breathing gets short and quick to take in more oxygen, your pulse and blood pressure skyrocket in order to get blood pumping to your muscles, your blood sugar spikes as your body tries to make more fuel available to you, and your digestion pauses so that the energy can go to more vital functions (like getting the eff out of dodge). Meanwhile, your body's HPA axis, which is the conglomeration of your hypothalamus, pituitary gland, and adrenal glands, produces cortisol to encourage your body to stay in beast mode for as long as possible. This fight-or-flight state is called "hyperarousal."

We're also biologically equipped with tools that can put out this fire-and-brimstone response. When the HPA axis believes the threat has passed, it stops producing cortisol and hands the reins over to the parasympathetic nervous system. The stress response begins to recede, the body returns to its comfortable, non-stressed resting state, and homeostasis is restored.

The only problem is that many of us get stuck in the hyperarousal state. This is thanks in large part to the fact that our brains perceive pretty much everything as stress—not just the original sources like natural predators or food scarcity that would have threatened our survival back in the day. Work deadlines, unexpected e-mails, traffic, negative emotions that arise after getting lost in your social media feed, fear of pandemics, fear and anxiety of the unknown—they all trigger the stress response. So do things like bacteria and viruses, environmental toxins, noise pollution, allergens, radiation, food allergies, processed food, sugar, alcohol, and chronic overstimulation.

It's no wonder that most of us are stuck when it comes to our stress setting.

How Does Stress Affect Sleep?

Hyperarousal is understood to be the main underlying factor in chronically disrupted sleep. It makes sense—if your brain and body are perpetually amped up, heated up, and chock-full of cortisol, there's no way that your sleep physiology can compete with that. Most people whose sleep is affected by stress are in a state of hyperarousal throughout the day. At night, this constant stress manifests as the inability to fall asleep or to get back to sleep after waking up in the middle of the night. This is then exacerbated by lying sleeplessly in bed with a restless mind, which often only becomes more anxious and stressed over the inability to sleep. Then lack of sleep becomes a stressor itself, making people even more reactive and vulnerable to stress, creating a vicious sleepless cycle.

Learning to Live (and Sleep) with Stress

You can't control external stressors. But you can control how you respond to them so that you can finally get off the adrenaline-cortisol roller coaster. The process begins with giving your body the support it needs to more seamlessly go with the flow. There's no one cure-all solution, and as Neil experienced in his own sleep-better journey, and as Frank sees with a majority of his patients, it takes a layered, long-term approach to healing how your body has been handling stress for what has been most likely a long time. The good news is that by assembling your sleep-better protocol, you'll be doing this on a daily basis. Here's what to focus on:

- **Practice relaxation techniques.** Meditation and deep breathing in particular can help you quiet hyperarousal not only before sleep but throughout the day, making it easier for you to find that calm, quiet baseline at bedtime. ("Breathe in Rhythm," page 113). In fact, go ahead and take ten deep breaths right now. We'll wait.
- **Move every day.** Consistent movement—including functional activities like gardening, walking the dog, and playing with your kids—not only helps to reduce stress but also provides its own sleep-supporting benefits. (Move to Sleep, page 102).

- **Find inner (digestive) peace.** Your diet and digestive health (especially your gut) play a large role in your state of mind and your ability to process stress. And things like sugar, processed food, and alcohol can fuel the hyperarousal fire by increasing inflammation and upsetting hormonal balance. All of the recommendations in Eat to Sleep (page 125) will help you create a calmer homeostatic baseline.

- **Find your rhythm.** One of the most effective things you can do to improve your stress management *and* your sleep is to finally get yourself back in rhythm—which is the name of the entire game, as far as we're concerned. Every step you take toward syncing yourself with nature's 24-hour sleep-wake cycle is one step closer to a lifetime of better nights and fewer stressed-out days.

DO THIS NOW

If you find yourself tossing and turning and not able to fall asleep within 20 to 30 minutes of going to bed, don't force it. Instead, turn to a relaxing, unstimulating activity like reading or writing in your journal—making sure to use low light ("Dim with the Dark," page 78)—or turn to any of the breathing exercises in "Breathe in Rhythm" (page 113) until you feel ready to wind down.

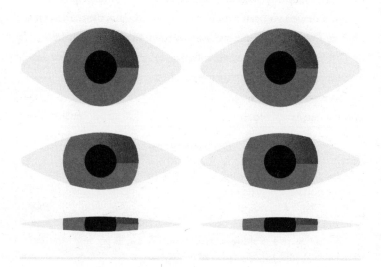

HAVE A POWERING-DOWN PRACTICE

Just like what you do all day long affects your sleep at night, how you wind down at the end of your day can make a difference in the quality and quantity of your rest. People think they can go 100 miles per hour then just stop and go to sleep. But that's not the way the body works— it's not a device you can simply switch off. Sleep is a *process,* with the body gradually responding to the setting sun, gently turning up the dial on its melatonin production, then coordinating the hundreds of metabolic processes all over the body that synchronize to help you get a good night's rest. Plus, the body thrives on consistency, preferring to know when exactly to shift into sleep mode each and every day. That's why one of the first things Frank recommends to his patients—and one of the greatest things you can do for your sleep—is to create a consistent practice for powering down in the evening.

Think of sleep as starting 60 to 90 minutes before you even get under the covers. This is the time when you're slowly taking your foot off the gas and then gently applying it to the brake. In other words, it's the time to move away from potentially stimulating activities and embrace calming, more sedative habits. It's definitely not the time to be watching something potentially upsetting on TV, hitting the treadmill, or sitting under full-blast overhead lighting. The goal is to support your sleep cycle by keeping your nervous system as chilled-out as possible. In fact, many of the recommended presleep rituals you see here are habits referenced elsewhere in this book because of their rest-promoting, rhythm-protecting potential.

Checklist for the Ideal Bedtime Practice

90 minutes before bed:

- Dim the lights (page 78).
- Switch your electronics to night mode and/or block blue light with glasses or a screen cover (page 79).
- Take a warm bath or shower (page 87).

60 minutes before bed:

- Turn off your electronics—and not just because of the melatonin-disrupting blue light (page 79). Just as your digestive system needs time to digest and metabolize the food you've eaten at dinner before you turn in for the night, your brain needs time to digest and metabolize the happenings of the day, which includes everything it's taking in from your phone, computer, and television.
- Start to entrain your nervous system to a slower beat. Put on some Bob Marley, take some CBD (page 158), and/or spend some time breathing in calming essential oils (page 198).

30 minutes before bed:

- Do some restorative movement (page 107), gentle stretching (page 107), and/or breathing exercises (page 113).
- Read a good book—a real one with pages.
- Go for the Big O (page 91).

TAKE A WARM BATH

This is one that gets tossed out there a lot when it comes to articles about how to sleep better. And we understand that it tends to get an eye roll because of its slightly unrealistic-seeming "indulgence" undertones. But taking a bath isn't reserved for people with spa-like bathrooms and the luxury of time. It's a scientifically proven method for encouraging the physiological processes that usher in sleep and increasing the amount of deep sleep you can get in a night. It also doesn't hurt that it's a pleasurable, relaxing activity that most people can find 20 to 30 minutes to do before bed.

Your temperature naturally dips at night, beginning about two hours before sleep. So when you mimic that decrease, you're prompting your brain to release melatonin and helping to reinforce your body's natural rhythm. A warm bath does just that (so does, to a lesser extent, a hot shower) by raising your core temperature a degree or two, then prompting a quick drop when you get out. That's because your dilated blood vessels send their extra heat radiating out into the air, leading to a steep decrease in your internal thermostat. And in turn, you may fall asleep more quickly and spend more time in deep sleep.

Your Nighttime Bath Rx

Take a bath one to two hours before bed (for some people, a bath can have the opposite effect when taken right before light's out) and soak for 20 to 30 minutes. Repeat as needed.

Additional supplements optional:

- **Epsom salts:** Their magnesium helps support your levels of GABA, a neurotransmitter that promotes sleep.
- **Essential oils:** These can relieve anxiety and stress, promote sleep, and generally smell nice. Check out the most relaxing varietals on page 197.
- **Dim, warm lighting:** Turn down to avoid melatonin disruption—there's a reason why a candlelit bath is so zen. See page 77 for our recommended sourcing guidelines.

SHUSH YOUR SNORING

Ideally, your breathing at night would be silent, quiet, and effortless, helping you drift into deep, restorative sleep. Snoring (and sleep apnea, which we'll talk more about in a moment) is not normal or healthy. While 40 percent of the adult population snores, if left unchecked, this could disrupt your nights and make you miss out on the essential benefits of REM sleep. Not to mention the fact that it's a major sound polluter in your sleep sanctuary and can also cause your partner to lose out on a restorative night's rest too.

Snoring is the result of air being obstructed while breathing at night. So the remedy is essentially to remove the obstruction, which, luckily for most people, can be done with relatively easy habit changes, changes in sleep posture, or by adopting snore-solution products and/or tech. Not all snorers are the same, so finding the answer for you might take some trial and error or mixing and matching.

IF YOU'RE NOT SURE WHETHER YOU SNORE

Most sleep-tracking apps and devices will let you know if you snore because of their audio sensors. You could also download the app SnoreLab, which listens specifically for snoring sounds and can record clips — in case you're still not convinced.

Your Snore-No-More Menu

- **Dietary changes:** Following the gut-healing recommendations in Eat to Sleep (page 125) and The Reset (page 225) can lead to weight loss and a decrease in inflammation, as well as a decrease in phlegm production—all of which can lead to the eradication of snoring.
- **Pass on that drink:** Alcohol causes body-wide relaxation, including your throat muscles, which can exacerbate snoring. Try not drinking for at least five hours before you go to bed.
- **Also pass on the pills:** Sleeping pills and sedatives have the same effect on snoring as alcohol.
- **Stop smoking:** It irritates the membranes in your nose and throat, which closes up the airways and makes snoring worse.
- **Give your mouth a workout:** Since snoring can be caused by muscular weakness in the mouth and throat, the apps Snorefree and SnoreGym use exercises for your lips, tongue, and throat to address the underlying imbalance and optimize airflow at night.
- **Get a raise:** Some people get relief by subtly raising their head to open their airways, either by adding a pillow or an adjustable base that can create a minor (but effective) incline in your mattress. These are nice, cost-effective alternatives to investing in a mattress that can be elevated on one side.
- **Shake things up:** New gadgets like the Smart Nora, ZEEQ Smart Pillow, and Philips SmartSleep Snoring Relief Band

detect snoring and either create gentle movement to prompt you to shift positions (the ZEEQ and Philips SmartSleep) or use a small pump to actually change the shape of your pillow to make that shift for you (Nora).

■ **Go old-school:** Nasal strips are sometimes enough to do the trick because they open your nasal passages and encourage more airflow. There are the classic, inexpensive adhesive versions you can find at most drugstores and then the slightly more expensive iterations that fit inside your nose, such as the Venyn Nose Vents.

An Important Note on Sleep Apnea

Snoring can be an indication that you have sleep apnea, a serious sleep disorder in which your breathing suddenly stops at night. While there are three types of sleep apnea, the most common is obstructive sleep apnea (OSA), which is a result of a restricted airway from the soft tissue and tongue in the back of the throat and compromised breathing through the nose. It's estimated that over 75 percent of severe OSA cases are undiagnosed and untreated, putting individuals at a high risk of heart attack, diabetes, stroke, congestive heart failure, impotence, reflux disease, insomnia, and respiratory disease, including Covid-19.

If you suspect that you suffer from OSA, we strongly recommend that you see a doctor for assessment and treatment. This can run the gamut from simple lifestyle changes (losing weight, avoiding alcohol, quitting smoking), to using CPAP (continuous positive airway pressure) therapy, to surgery, to cutting-edge facial "gear" that's espoused by a specialty field called epigenetic orthodontics.

GET MORE VITAMIN O

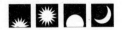

Sleep isn't the only thing the bed is for—sex and self-pleasure also warrant a spot under the covers. That's not just because it makes sense from a logistical perspective; there's ample research indicating that orgasm is beneficial for sleep on a number of levels. This is mainly a result of your brain, nervous system, adrenals, and pituitary glands releasing the following doozy of a feel-good hormone cocktail after the big O:

Oxytocin, aka the "love hormone," is released when we do intimate physical things with each other—hugging, touching, having sex. Its levels are increased through orgasm, which has a calming effect, decreasing cortisol and paving the way for melatonin to do its thing and produce deep sleep.

Serotonin is critical for producing melatonin and maintaining normal sleep-wake cycles. It's also responsible for increasing deep, non-REM sleep.

Norepinephrine is a hormone and neurotransmitter that parts of the nervous system use to balance the overall stress response in the body and regulate the sleep cycle. It too is involved in the synthesis of melatonin and is notably released during REM sleep. Cycling between REM and non-REM sleep is a crucial part of the body's nocturnal process, which is largely due to the yin-yang relationship between serotonin and norepinephrine.

Prolactin is linked to sexual pleasure, but levels of this hormone are also naturally higher when we sleep, suggesting that an extra dose before bed does the body good. But there's a caveat: The amount of prolactin you produce is intrinsically linked to the quality of your orgasm and sexual satisfaction. Men produce four times more prolactin when having an orgasm through intercourse versus through masturbation, and women also see increased levels when their needs are more satisfactorily met. That said, the sleep-bettering, immune-system-strengthening, quality-of-life-boosting benefits of prolactin are favorable whether you're reaping them with a partner or solo.

Vasopressin gets injected directly into the brain after sex and, along with oxytocin, contributes to your overall feeling of *aaaaah*. Like oxytocin, it's a hormone that plays a role in bonding, sexual motivation, and mitigating the response to stress, and it too decreases the levels of cortisol to help pave the way for sleep and increased sleep quality.

Better Sex for Better Sleep

Having an orgasm can be a full-on sedative for most people, so we encourage you to "take your sleep-aid supplement" during your pre-bed practice (page 86). But just like you can't cut corners like popping a pill to get great sleep, getting the best possible benefits from sex with a partner requires some effort. Consider it the most fun homework you could have.

- **Communicate.** Intimacy isn't only physical; it's emotional. For many people, sexual satisfaction is only possible when they feel emotionally connected with their partners. Make sure that both of you feel heard, supported, and safe in your relationship as well as your sexual space.
- **Move more.** Having a regular movement practice (page 102) not only boosts circulation and energy levels (key ingredients

for better sex), it also awakens sensitivity in your body, which leads to a greater desire to do the deed.

- **Get in rhythm.** The name of the game here! Having sex at night is physiologically beneficial and is also what we're culturally programmed to do, but from a biological perspective, 11 p.m. is pretty much the worst time to have sex. It's when we're least likely to be hormonally aroused and most of us are exhausted after a long day. As you fine-tune your pre-bed ritual, consider moving sex up on the timeline.

- **Get better sleep.** We know, we know—that's kind of the whole point of all this. But sleep deprivation is the number-one mood killer because when you're out of energy, your body isn't interested in what it considers to be nonessential activities. Also, as you saw in "The Out-of-Rhythm Body" (page 26), not sleeping well tanks the production of libido-boosting hormones. So if you're not feeling frisky right out of the gate, don't pressure yourself or your partner to have sex for sex's sake. Follow some of the biggies from your sleep-better protocol (eating in rhythm, syncing with the sun, following a consistent sleep schedule), and after a couple weeks you'll see your desire and orgasmic potential start to ignite.

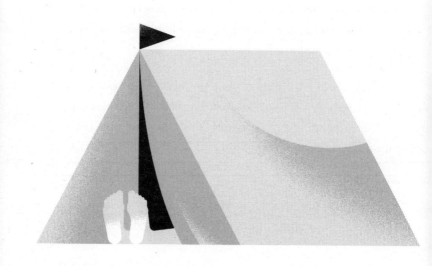

GO BACK TO NATURE

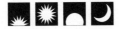

It's not an accident that our body is governed by rhythm. There are cyclical elements to everything in nature—the sun rises and sets, the tides ebb and flow, the seasons turn, creatures live and die. As Chinese medicine teaches, our microcosm (our internal body) is a direct reflection of the macrocosm (our external environment). Our biology is directly influenced by our surroundings, imprinting and entraining to the beat it hears. But when we're distanced from Mother Nature, we are also distanced from our Mother Rhythm. Even though it might seem like we're in constant contact with the elements (we can see the sky, feel the breeze, know what season it is), our modern lifestyle has us very far removed. We can wake and sleep independently from the sun, have no need to be out foraging for food, and spend most of our time in buildings that insulate us from all things outdoors. While this has been a major upgrade for us in many ways, it's the underlying cause of why so many of us have slipped out of sync.

If you're on a quest to reset that rhythm, then the ultimate place to go looking for it is where it all started in the first place. The closer we get to nature, the more in sync we get, the more our health improves, the more our sleep improves, and the better our health stays. Aside from getting out into the natural sunlight during the day ("Sync with the Sun," page 74), there are a few significant ways you can go back to your Master Clock roots:

- **Shift with the Seasons:** Modern life is essentially seasonless. The demands of our climate-controlled lives don't take into account the shifting temperatures, energies, and rhythms that unfold every few months. But in traditional Chinese medicine and other traditional healing practices, tuning in to the seasons is the foundation for bringing someone back into balance. Because as our environments change, so do our bodies' needs. Think about the newfound warmth of the spring, how energized it makes you feel, your desire to eat fresh, succulent produce; versus winter, when your body all but begs for the coziest sweaters, midday naps, and warming, hearty meals. That's the pull of the seasons, which we sometimes honor in small ways but, for the most part, tend to ignore.

When you understand the characteristics of the seasons, you better understand how to bring yourself into rhythm with them. We recommend fine-tuning your habits with the seasons—how you eat and move, and of course, how you sleep. Think about embracing the dynamic spirit of spring and summer, choosing more rigorous activities during the day, and taking advantage of the body's increased ability to digest raw foods by filling your meals with a bounty of seasonal produce. With the longer, sun-filled days, it's natural to stay up a bit later to take advantage (and we give you permission to do so). In the fall and winter, turn inwards. Think about how you can restore your body and mind with gentle movement and reflection, and give yourself deep, fortifying nourishment with slow-cooked meals from foods like root vegetables, which pull their nutrients from deep in the ground. We also encourage you to take advantage of the shorter, darker days and get a touch more sleep.

A helpful tool to smooth the transition between seasons is doing The Reset as the seasons change, especially between winter and spring, and again between summer and fall.

- **Feel the Earth Move:** Aside from the benefits of things like fresh air and natural light, the Earth itself also provides its own daily dose of sleep-supportive medicine. When you physically make contact with the planet's surface, you are, in effect, reconnecting your internal electrical system to the Earth's power grid. Current thinking (get it?) is that when you take off your shoes and stand on the ground (or lie on the grass or walk on the beach), you are harnessing the natural negative electrical charge of the Earth. Owing to emerging research, we now know that this has a number of benefits, including promoting anti-inflammatory activity by neutralizing positively charged free radicals, improving energy levels, reducing stress and anxiety, reducing headaches (both hormone- and tension-related), increasing endurance, shortening healing and recovery times, and reducing the effects of jet lag.[43] But most noteworthy for our purposes is that it also regulates your biorhythms, primarily by resynchronizing cortisol to its proper patterns.[44] So by restoring the balance of your body's bioelectric motherboard, you're also resetting your sleep-wake cycle.

  The simplest method for getting grounded, or "earthing" as its commonly called, is to stand or walk barefoot directly on the earth, whether it's dirt, grass, or sand (or concrete, to a lesser extent). Try to do this a few times a week, or whenever you can, and for a minimum of 30 minutes, as it takes at least half an hour to access meaningful health benefits. For extra credit, consider giving The Ultimate Synchronizer meditation (page 116) a shot. If that's not possible, you could also invest in earthing gadgets, such as grounding mats or bed pads, which effectively deliver similar bioelectric feedback that can positively affect your body's natural internal electrical stability and rhythms.

- **Camp Out:** Research has found that just two days spent entirely outdoors can substantially shift your internal clock to sync with an optimal sleep–wake cycle.[45] First, there's the consistent exposure to natural light and true, total darkness. Then there's the dipping nighttime temperatures signaling for increased melatonin and nighttime repair mode. And, perhaps most importantly, there's less access to—and need for—cell service (and by extension, no artificial blue light or overly stimulated mental chatter). The Great Outdoors is basically the ultimate sleep chamber. If you are struggling with significant and chronic sleep issues, consider packing up your gear (or borrowing a friend's) and heading out of town for the weekend.

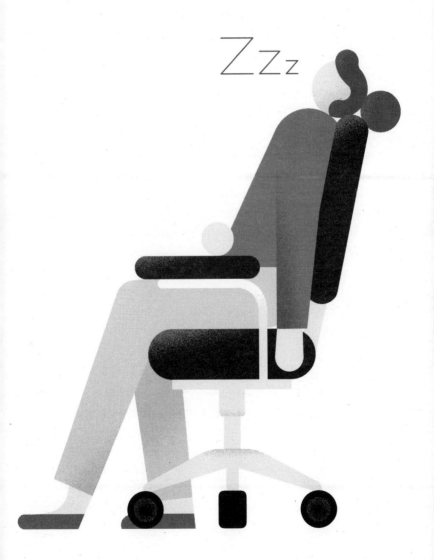

ZZz

TO NAP OR NOT TO NAP?

Napping can be a polarizing topic in the sleep world. On one hand, naps are a great way to catch up on sleep if you're deprived. Some experts believe that it doesn't matter when we sleep so long as we get enough total shut-eye hours since, according to them, we were never meant to sleep in one long stretch. And many warm-weather cultures observe the siesta, a 60- to 90-minute nap between 2 p.m. and 4 p.m.

On the other hand, napping can be a notorious nighttime sleep-stealer, making it more difficult to fall asleep and stay there. We like to think of naps as just another tool in your rhythm-resetting toolbox—they can be beneficial, but you have to be smart about how you use them.

Let's go back to the brain for a minute. Adenosine is a chemical that the brain produces simply because it's awake. The longer you're awake, the more adenosine that accumulates in the brain. And all that accumulated adenosine eventually builds up and makes you and your brain sleepy at the appropriate evening time. This is called "sleep pressure."

As anyone who has curled up on the sofa on a rainy afternoon can tell you, napping relieves sleep pressure. However, by prematurely doing so in the middle of the day instead of at night, you can potentially interfere with your natural sleep-wake cycle. If you're someone who tends to struggle with falling asleep at night, napping may not be for you.

But for others, a nap can be a powerful sleep supplement. Research has shown that a well-timed, well-executed nap can boost alertness, mood, and productivity. One particularly fascinating study looked at the effects that a short nap had on the afternoon training session of athletes who were suffering from some degree of sleep loss. After a quick 30-minute snooze, both their performance and mental sharpness improved compared to teammates who didn't get to take a rest.[46]

The Three-Step Quickie

1. **Choose the right time:** Your body temperature naturally dips between 2 p.m. and 4 p.m., causing a small uptick in melatonin and a subtle downshift in your energy. (Yes, the post-lunch slump is real.) Aim to nap during this window or slightly earlier; anything later will most likely mess with bedtime.

2. **Keep it short.★** The most potent naps are brief—even 10 to 20 minutes can boost your alertness and mental function without leaving you feeling drowsy. Cap your naps at 30 minutes.

> **★The Long-Nap Exception**
>
> Naps longer than 30 minutes are called for in situations where nighttime sleep is being regularly disturbed, such as for parents of a newborn. In these cases, giving your body the rest it needs at any time in the day and for any length of time is more beneficial than not.

3. **Repeat.** There's evidence that consistent nappers reap more benefits than dabblers, so consider making regular napping a habit.

TRY A "NAPPACCINO"

While we can't take credit for the clever name, we can pass along this suggestion, which has been doing the rounds on the sleep circuit and is backed up by anecdotal evidence. The Nappaccino calls for drinking an 8-ounce cup of coffee *before* you take a nap. That way you're not only heading off the drowsy-making adenosine build-up that caffeine contributes to, you're also waking up just as the caffeine is kicking in, 20 to 25 minutes later. In theory then, you're reaping double-whammy energy-boosting benefits.

CHAPTER 5

MOVE TO SLEEP

We are designed to move—and not just from the car to the desk to the house to the couch. Regular movement *all day long* is part of our genetic code, and because of that, our wellness depends on it. Moving your body improves everything: your metabolism, your microbiome, your immunity, your stress response, your mood, and most notably, your body rhythms and your sleep. This is why incorporating an intentional movement practice (or exercising, or working out, or whatever you'd like to call it), in addition to getting your body up and about throughout the day, is one of our sleep-better recommendations.

Simply put, people who regularly exercise and sit for fewer than eight hours a day sleep better than those who don't. Scientific evidence indicates that exercise can be an effective natural therapy for insomnia and can decrease the severity of sleep-disordered breathing such as sleep apnea. And exercise increases total sleep time and slow-wave (or deep) sleep. Here is why:

- **Exercise increases your body's amount of adenosine,** the drowsy-inducing chemical that creates "sleep pressure," or the natural biological urge to sleep. This helps regulate circadian rhythm.

- **Exercise temporarily raises your core body temperature,** which then causes an equal and opposite reaction: decreased body temperature at night. This helps encourage deeper sleep cycles.
- **Exercise triggers the release of cortisol,** which, when timed correctly during your day, encourages the hormone's natural rise and retreat that your body needs to sleep at night.

What Exercise Is Best for Sleep?

Short answer: Whatever you'll do on a regular basis. Longer answer: Both aerobic exercise, such as running, cycling, and high-intensity interval training (HIIT), and resistance training, including weightlifting, resistance bands, yoga, and Pilates, have been found to deliver sleep-promoting benefits—as long as they're done consistently.

How Intense Does Exercise Have to Be for Me to See Benefits?

Not very. Even gentle activities like walking can help. Researchers found that middle-aged men who adopted a walking regimen were able to increase their self-rated sleep quality during a month-long study.[47] More important than intensity is how much activity you're getting every day. That same study concluded that the more minutes participants spent moving, the better they rated their sleep overall.

How Much Exercise Do I Need for Better Sleep?

There is no exact number specific to sleep, but moving more for your health is going to get you the results you want. Your ideal amount will vary depending on things like your age and fitness level, but a good, simple start is to aim for 30 minutes of moderate aerobic exercise, five days a week. But as a general rule of thumb, just move *more,* all day, every day. The less sedentary you are, the better you'll sleep at night.

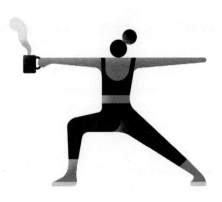

EXERCISE IN RHYTHM

As vast and numerous as the benefits of intentional exercise are (which we're differentiating from functional, everyday movement), unlocking its sleep-supporting power depends on whether you're using it to support your sleep-wake cycle. Remember, what you do during the day and evening sets the stage for how well you'll rest at night, namely because of the 24-hour chain reaction of events happening in your body from the time you wake up in the morning. Your habits throughout the day either support this rhythm and keep it running steady, or throw it off course.

It's no different for exercise. You want the *time of day* you're exerting yourself and the *type of movement* you're doing to reinforce your body's innate rhythm, not be at odds with it. For Neil, this was a big piece of the puzzle. He didn't have a consistent workout routine (issue one), and when he did get to the gym for a sweaty, high-intensity session, it was after 6 p.m. (issue two). Working with Frank, he got the nudge he needed to move daily—even if it was just a walk outside during a break between meetings—while shifting his tougher workouts to earlier in the day.

When to Keep It Upbeat

In order to figure out how to use moderate- to high-intensity exercise as a sleep-encouraging tool, it's helpful to understand what exactly this type of exercise is: a stressor. When you get in a good, sweaty workout, you're actually inflicting minor damage on your body. You're creating microtears in your muscle fibers, which then elevates your stress hormones, your inflammatory biomarkers, and even your blood sugar. This temporary and beneficial stress (also known as hormesis) prompts your body to repair, which it does as you sleep. (Another reason why getting a good night's rest is important—it helps you reap the rewards of your workout.)

But if you're triggering that stress response right before you go to bed and flushing your body with the cortisol that it's working to lower for the night, it's going to interfere with your sleep. Moderate- to high-intensity exercise also releases a big dose of feel-good dopamine and endorphins, which make you feel alert. Lastly, this type of exercise raises your core body temperature, which can take as long as four to six hours to come back down again. If your body is trying to lower its temperature in preparation for sleep, then that temporary spike is going to hinder that process.

The Moderate- to High-Intensity Exercise Rx

Move in the morning. Counter to what most people assume—that if you tire yourself out on the treadmill at night, you'll tire yourself out for sleep—working out in the morning is ideal if you want to sleep better at night. A recent study showed that exercisers who worked out at 7 a.m. slept longer and had 75 percent more time in the reparative deep-sleep stage than those who worked out at lunchtime or in the evening.[48] Getting a cortisol spike in the morning not only helps your energy and productivity—more effectively than that cup of coffee—it also puts your cortisol rhythm on target to steadily drop throughout the day, reaching its lowest levels when it's time to sleep.

Or have a cardio curfew. Depending on your chronotype (page 71), you may feel a second surge of energy in the afternoon that you like to take advantage of in order to work out. This too can be strategic for sleep, especially because the initial uptick in your core temperature will be waning just as you're, literally, chilling out for the night. Your post-workout temperature cooldown tends to dip slightly below your normal thermostat, which is perfect bedtime conditions.

If you do prefer to work out in the afternoon—or it's your only option given your schedule—aim to wrap up four to six hours before you plan to be asleep. This will give your body enough time to cool down, your parasympathetic nervous system the opportunity to recalibrate after the influx of cortisol, and your brain a chance to wind down after riding its endorphin and dopamine high.

If evening is the only time you can work out: Consider choosing gentler, low-impact activities such as yoga, Tai Chi, Pilates, or a walk. These activities won't ramp up your body and brain and are beneficial for ushering in sleep, which you'll read more about below.

It's also worth pointing out that some people's sleep is not affected by what time of day they exercise. Exercising at night can actually benefit how quickly some people drift off. That's perfectly normal. Our tips here are conservative recommendations based on solving a general sleep issue. Once you've reset your rhythm, you may find that when you get in a workout doesn't ultimately make a difference.

When to Slow It Down

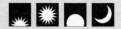

Restorative movement, or low-intensity movement that's deeply relaxing for the body, is a subtle but powerful tool in anyone's sleep kit. Frank regularly encourages his clients to adopt these kinds of practices—no matter why they've come to see him—because of the wide-ranging beneficial effects they have on your body and your health. At Frank's suggestion, Neil started incorporating Iyengar yoga into his routine, which not only helped chill him out but also reduced aches and pains both during and after working out.

But contrary to what you might assume about slow and gentle exercises, like restorative yoga, Tai Chi, stretching, and a leisurely walk, they aren't only meant for your pre-bed ritual (though they do work best at this time—more on that in a moment). In addition to supporting your more intense workouts as a harmonizing yin to high-intensity yang that can set you up for quicker recovery, fewer injuries, and less-sore muscles, restorative movement has the ability to soothe a frazzled sympathetic nervous system and improve your stress response.

As a rule of thumb, restorative movement is something that feels relaxing and doesn't get your heart rate up too much. Some examples include:

going for a walk

Tai Chi

Qigong

yoga (restorative or yin, not anything ultra-demanding and
sweaty)

foam rolling and stretching (more on page 123)

Your brain is constantly being informed about how your body is feeling, thanks to its network of sensory neurons. Your brain usually takes your body's lead, so if your muscles are tense and your breathing is short and shallow, then your brain goes into stress mode, pumping out cortisol to keep you on high alert. Over the course of the day, we naturally build up tension just going about our business, and if not released properly, we head to bed with, quite literally, a head full of stress.

When you can release that tension, relax your muscles, and deepen your breath by practicing restorative movement, you're not only creating a more relaxed physical state, you're also creating a more relaxed mental state, as well as a perfectly calibrated neurochemistry that encourages better sleep.

The beauty of restorative exercise is that you don't have to wait until the evening to reap its sleep-boosting benefits. These movements have a cumulative effect because they help to continuously keep your sympathetic nervous system in check and your cortisol levels exactly where they need to be. Restorative exercises, including stretching and yoga postures, provide different benefits at different times:

First thing in the morning: Restorative movement gently
energizes the body and boosts mental alertness, especially if
you're feeling a little foggy from a not-so-great night's sleep.
Engaging in just a few minutes of restorative exercise will help
get you back on track, instead of derailing your day's rhythm
the way too much caffeine or sugary snacks would.

Late afternoon: Around 3 p.m., when you hit the post-lunch slump, restorative movement can provide the same benefits as that cup of coffee you'd normally go for—without putting a damper on your sleep later that evening.

Evening: As part of your pre-bed routine, these gentle movements put your mind at ease, steady your breath, and reduce muscle tension without getting your heart rate up. They create the perfect conditions for you and your body to receive sleep.

Instant Chill Pills

The following restorative poses have been part of Frank's "prescriptions" for patients for years and are particularly helpful in the evening just before bed to power down. Just a short time spent in these poses is the ultimate sleep send-off, not to mention a great way to fend off night-time wake-ups caused by pain or cramping (more on that on page 139):

Seated Forward Bend with Chair

This modified version of *janu shirshasana* ensures that you can rest your forehead (and third eye) on a soft surface, thereby fully activating the relaxing benefits of the stretch. Sit on the ground or a mat with your legs stretched out in front of your body. Arrange a chair in front of you so that you'll be able to comfortably rest your head on its seat. You will want to pad it a bit with a folded towel or blanket. Bend your right leg in toward your chest and then open the right hip so that the right foot connects to the inside of your left leg close to the groin. Reach forward toward your left leg to stretch, resting your head on the chair and your arms on your left shin or ankle. You don't want to feel too much strain in your leg. Stay in this position for up to 30 seconds total. Then slowly lift your arms up and repeat on the right side.

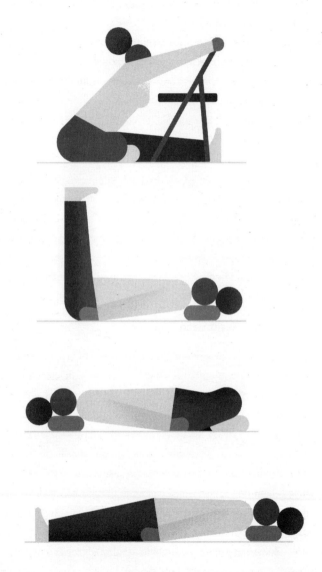

Modified Supta Baddha Konasana

Also known as "Goddess Pose," this posture only takes about five minutes to generate a strong beneficial effect that calms the breathing and softens the emotional center of the chest. It also comes in handy after meals to soothe digestion, if that's an issue for you.

Before you get comfortable, grab a yoga bolster, sofa cushion (a rectangular one from the back), or two neatly folded towels or blankets. You'll also want an additional blanket folded in thirds, or another towel folded the same. You might also want additional towels or blankets to use as additional supports, especially if you have tight hips.

Sit on the floor with loosely crossed legs. Snuggle the short edge of your cushion up against your sacrum (or butt). Lie back and place the folded blanket or towel under your head for support. Your head should be higher than your heart, and your chin parallel to the floor, not tipping up to the ceiling or down to your chest. If your knees are hovering above the ground, feel free to tuck the extra blankets or towels under each knee so your legs can completely relax. You'll know when you've hit the mark on your supports—your whole body will feel blissfully "held" and relaxed. (We're sleepy just writing about it.)

Melt into this posture for about 10 to 15 minutes, watching as your breath moves in and out of your body. Don't force your breath, just notice that it's flowing.

Legs Up the Wall

This do-anywhere pose regulates blood pressure, refreshes the abdominal organs, and encourages circulation (for some people, it can even offer relief from varicose veins).

First, locate a blanket or towel you can use to cushion your bum and/or head, along with a wall that has an unobstructed bit of floor in front of it. Sit with your side to the wall with your knees bent so that your left hip is pressed up against the wall. Slowly roll onto your back so that your tush is right up against the wall with both feet just above. Extend your feet straight so that your body forms an L, keeping your bottom as close to the wall as your hamstrings will allow. Make sure your chin stays parallel to the floor, not tipping up to the ceiling or pressing down to your chest.

Extend your arms to your side and bend them at the elbows 90 degrees so that they're making a "cactus" shape. Relax your head, face, neck, shoulders, and belly. Breathe as you hang out for 10 to 15 minutes. As a variation, you can spread your legs into a gentle V on the wall. To come out, bring your knees back into your chest and roll to one side.

Note: It's normal to feel a slight tingling in your legs. But if it becomes painful, bring your legs down and take an easy cross-legged position with your legs still resting on the wall.

Savasana

Also known as "corpse pose," this closing posture for your practice helps seal in all that relaxing work you just did. Lie flat on your back on the floor or bed, comfortably. Keep your eyes closed and separate your feet about a foot apart. Keep your arms out by your sides, with palms facing up. With eyes closed, silently instruct your body to relax.

Slowly move your attention to each part of your body, from your left foot to your left leg and then move your way to the right foot and leg, followed by your hips, abdomen, chest, hands, arms, and each part of your head.

Focus on imagining and relaxing all of your organs—your brain, lungs, heart, stomach, kidneys, colon, bladder.

Bring your attention to all of your five senses (sight, sound, smell, touch, taste), which will automatically start to surrender.

Finally, begin to observe your own mind without attaching to any particular thought, but rather allowing thoughts to arise and melt away.

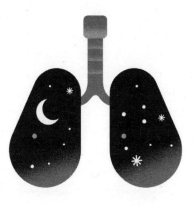

BREATHE IN RHYTHM

If there could be another title for this book, it might easily be *Wired and Tired: The Story of Your Life*. That pretty much sums up almost everyone who walks into Frank's office—including Neil—and it's a mental and physical state that is at the root of a number of chronic conditions today. Many of us are walking around amped up from stress all day long, and then can't turn off that switch when it's time to go to sleep at night. As a result, our sleep suffers, leading to more stress, less sleep, and on it goes. So we end up exhausted but unable to relax. But you won't find the solution at the bottom of a bottle of Xanax or wine. Instead, the (side effect-free) answer to your problem is in your breath.

Meditation and breath work are two of the most effective tools we have when it comes to actively turning off the stress response and turning on the relaxation response. Changing how you breathe and where you're focusing your mind can physically reprogram the brain via the vagus nerve, the ethernet cord connecting the brain and the body. Just as a tense body and short, shallow breaths can trigger the brain into thinking it's in trouble ("Loosen Up," page 120), a calm body and deep, slow breaths do just the opposite. It tells the brain that we're safe, and calls forth the release of GABA, an anti-anxiety neurotransmitter that promotes a sense of serenity and ease.

In addition to promoting the kind of adaptability and resilience that are necessary if you're going to be able to handle the endless waves of stress that life will bring (and yes, life will bring endless waves of stress; "Stop Stressing about Stress," page 80), meditation and breath work give your brain a workout, improving attention, memory, processing speed, and creativity. These activities may also counteract age-related atrophying that can lead to cognitive conditions like dementia. But most notably for our purposes:

Meditation and breath work decrease blood pressure and decrease stress and anxiety, essentially "priming the pump" for easier sleep onset at night.

They have been shown to increase sleep time, improve sleep quality, and make it easier to fall (and stay) asleep, mostly owing to the fact that they reduce hyperarousal in the brain.

They create physiological changes that are similar to the early phases of sleep — a slowed pulse, lowered blood pressure, and decreased stress hormones.

They have been found to be as effective as a prescription drug in some individuals with insomnia, without the side-effects.[49]

They can be used with other sleep techniques such as cognitive behavioral therapy for insomnia (CBT-I), which has been shown to improve sleep better than CBT-I alone.

Meditation Do's

Do observe your circadian rhythm when choosing when and how to meditate. While most meditation styles feel relaxing, as you hone your practice, you'll find that many approaches to mindfulness are meant to create a sharp, alert mind. That's why a true meditation (versus deep breathing exercises) is best done in the morning or at least a few hours before bed. There are also mindfulness and breathing practices that are meant to help you tune out and drift to sleep (we've included some on pages 118–119). Both methods will ultimately help you sleep better at night. Just be sure to pick the practice that best fits the time of day you intend to meditate.

Do aim for a minimum of 10 to 15 minutes a day. No month-long retreats required to reap the benefits.

Do find a style that works for you. We've included some simple exercises to start with, but there are many different meditation techniques, styles, and philosophies (Transcendental, Kundalini, Vedic, Zen Buddhist, to name a few). We encourage you to shop around, try a few, and see what resonates with you.

Do explore apps like Headspace, Calm, Aura, Insight Timer, and 10 percent Happier for personalized, inexpensive guidance.

TUNE IN AND TURN ON FOR THE DAY

Many meditation experts will tell you that the purest aim of the practice is to fully awaken, focus, and energize the mind, making the following exercises better suited for earlier in the day. Although you should reach for these in the morning after you wake up or any time in the afternoon when you find yourself needing to re-center, they are still actively supporting your journey toward sleep. They completely relax the body, returning it to an even-keeled baseline. That ultimately helps keep your sympathetic nervous system and cortisol levels in check, making it easier to fall asleep at night. Here are a couple of meditation practices to get you started:

The Basic Model: Simple Seated Meditation

Time: 10 minutes

- Choose a quiet and comfortable spot that is free of distractions.
- Set a timer for 10 minutes.
- Take a comfortable seated position. You can sit cross-legged on the floor, or you can sit in a chair. If you are sitting on the floor, you may want to use a cushion so your hips are raised. Keep your spine straight and tall.
- Choose an object to concentrate on. It could be a mantra such as *Om* (considered to be the original vibration and sound of the universe), *I am peaceful* (or other reassuring thought to anchor yourself to), or an uplifting image such as a full moon or a flower.
- Now begin paying attention to your breath as you inhale and exhale. The purpose of this practice is not to control the breath or slow it down but simply to bring your awareness to your breathing. You can feel the sensation of the breath around your nostrils.
- During your practice, your attention will wander away from the breath. This is not a problem—it doesn't mean you're doing anything wrong. Simply note that your attention has wandered and bring your focus back to your breath as you inhale and as you exhale.

The Ultimate Synchronizer: Meditation with Nature

Time: 15 to 30 minutes

- Find a park, woods, beach, nature preserve, or reservoir. In a pinch you can do this in your home or apartment and tune into the details of the space.
- If you can, take off your shoes.

- Begin to forget anything that happened earlier today before this practice. Try not to anticipate what happens next.
- Begin walking for a few minutes until you come to a place where you feel like pausing. When you arrive there, stop.
- Stand still for a moment and take in your surroundings. Notice where you are. Take note of everything—the trees, grass, sand, water, sounds, the texture of the air. Take 10 deep breaths, inhaling through the nose and exhaling through the mouth.
- After a few more breaths, allow your feet to become more sensitive to what they are touching—grass, rocks, sand. Feel where your weight is. Maybe it is more over your heels. Maybe you are leaning forward slightly.
- Notice how your body feels. What feels sticky, tired, achy? Which parts feel loose and easy? Take five more breaths, directing the breath to the sticky places. If your hips feel tight, inhale, picture the breath traveling down and into the hips, then exhale, picturing the tension and pain streaming out of the hip socket. Likewise, if your shoulders feel as if they are rolled forward, inhale, bringing the breath into the shoulder socket, and exhale, imagining the shoulders easing back into their sockets, the shoulder blades sliding down the back.
- With this newfound spaciousness, begin walking again. For the remaining minutes allow yourself to be completely absorbed by what is in front of you, beside you, under you, behind you. Look at the bark on the trees, the stones in the sand, a spiderweb, a flower's pistil, the shape of seaweed, the shape of your footprint, the length of your stride. Become sensitive to where the air is meeting your skin—maybe on your face and hands. Let yourself be curious about everything. If you wonder what is under a rock, look. If you are curious about a kind of tree, move in closer and study it. If you wonder about an animal, stop and watch it. Listen for the wind, the birds, your breath.

- When you are done, notice how you feel. Maybe your breath is easier. Maybe you are more relaxed. Maybe you feel more connected.

DROP OUT FOR THE NIGHT

Unwinding for bed calls for slowing your breath and climbing deep inside the coziest parts of yourself. The best way to do this is with easy breathing practices or guided meditations that focus on relaxation and letting go of the day. (The apps listed on page 115 are particularly great resources for the latter.) Here are a couple to get you started, which hopefully you'll add to your powering-down practice (page 91):

The Speedy Soother: Abdominal Breathing Basics

Time: 10 to 30 minutes

- Find a quiet spot where you won't be disturbed. Get into a relaxed position, whether lying down or sitting up.
- Put your hands on your abdomen, gently close your mouth, and touch your tongue to your upper palate. Begin to breathe through your nose. If your nose is blocked for any particular reason, it is fine to breathe through your mouth.
- Inhale deeply and slowly into your abdomen (rather than your chest), being aware of your diaphragm moving downward and your abdomen expanding. Your hands on your abdomen will feel the expansion like a balloon filling.
- At the end of the inhalation, don't hold the breath; exhale slowly, so that your abdomen falls automatically as you exhale.

- Try to get all the breath out of your lungs on the expiration. The expiration should normally be about twice as long as the inhalation when you get relaxed.
- Keep repeating this, keeping your focus on your hands rising on the abdomen with inhalation and falling as you exhale.

The Tension Terminator: Abdominal Breathing Advanced

Time: 10 to 30 minutes

- Find a comfortable position. Do 10 abdominal breaths as described previously.
- Then imagine with your next inhalation that you are breathing into a tense area such as a tight neck, a strained lower back, your head, your buttocks, or wherever you may feel pain or tension.
- With the exhalation, let the tension go out of your nose along with the air.
- Keep repeating this until the pain or tension starts to ease.

GIVE GRATITUDE

A growing body of research shows that by giving a little thanks for what you have in your life you can reap the benefits of decreased stress, decreased symptoms of depression, decreased risk of heart disease, and better sleep. (And reduced materialism and increased generosity among adolescents, so consider getting the whole family involved.) Before or after your evening breathing session, take a moment to write down one thing you're grateful for (preferably with pen and paper in low lighting, not on your phone). It can be big and lofty, such as all the love you experience in your household. Or it can be a small victory, like appreciating how well you made dinner that night. Every so often, take a moment to look through past entries and appreciate your riches.

LOOSEN UP

One of the biggest complaints Frank hears from his patients (especially those who are on the more seasoned end of the spectrum) is that their aches and pains wake them in the night. Stiff backs, stiff joints, stiff necks—it all adds up to a less restful night's sleep. Many people blame it on their mattress. That could perhaps be the case (and should be ruled out; see how to do this in "Make Your Bed," page 182), but more likely it's coming from somewhere else, usually your own body.

Our everyday lives are basically a recipe for tight muscles and achy joints. We spend most of our time sitting (a hip-tightening posture that wreaks havoc on the back), hunched over our devices (there go the neck and shoulders), and generally tensing as we're bombarded with a variety of stressors (real and perceived). These small insults add up to a body that is increasingly stiff and riddled with aches and pains. That's not good for your sleep, and it's definitely not good for your health.

Aside from causing discomfort as you try to settle in for the night, this kind of physical tension is translated by the brain as mental tension. In fact, the brain interprets a stiff, rigid body as an indication that the body might not be safe, and that it *shouldn't* relax. And an amped-up, stressed-out mind is the last thing you want when it comes to sleep (or anything else, for that matter).

One way to hit the pressure release valve is to gently stretch your muscles at night and again in the morning, after your body may have gotten stiff. Releasing the tension held in hot spots like your hips, neck, chest, and shoulders signals to your brain that it can drop its guard, submit, and snooze. It's the perfect addition to your powering-down routine (page 91).

NON-RX MUSCLE RELAXER

Adding Epsom salts to your warm evening bath (page 88) is an effective way to relieve tight muscles, a result of their natural magnesium content. The mineral is also helpful for promoting sleep!

Aaahmazing Tension Dissolvers

Couch Stretch

This supported stretch helps to open up hip flexors that get shortened the more we sit, which can create a "pulling" effect on the lower back.

- Stand in front of your sofa, facing away from it. Bend your left leg and rest your left knee slightly behind you on the sofa.
- Stand tall as you squeeze your butt and abs. Hold the position for two minutes (you won't like it very much, but that means it's doing its job).
- Switch and repeat on the other leg.

Note: If you find this position challenging and want to make it a bit easier on yourself, move your bent knee away from the sofa. The farther away your knee is, the less severe the stretch. Work up gradually until you're doing the full stretch.

Piriformis Stretch

Also known as the "figure four," this is one of the best stretches for releasing all the tightness we hold in our hips—the epicenter of tension. This reduces the strain on the lower back and is great for alleviating back pain and sciatica as well as improving hip mobility.

- Sit toward the front of a chair seat so that the edge just hits the intersection of your butt muscles and hamstrings.
- Cross your right ankle over the left knee so that the ankle bone rests on the soft flesh just above the knee. Flex the right foot.
- Lengthen your spine, making the sides of your body longer, and then lean slightly forward with this extended spine. Breathe deeply. You should feel the stretch deep in your butt muscles. Hold for one to two minutes, moving the torso closer to the legs as the hip opens. Switch sides.

Note: Avoid rounding the spine; keep the back flat and imagine hinging forward from the hips.

Ultimate Neck and Shoulder Release

The name says it all. This stretch is ideal for letting go of all the emotional and physical burdens we put on this part of our body and will help you release tight upper back, neck, and shoulder muscles. You'll need two tennis balls.

- Lie on your back, knees bent and feet hip-width apart so that your kneecaps are in line with your hip bones. Place two tennis balls at the top of your shoulder blades, side by side, in the area where you would love to have a massage. Slowly lower your head and shoulders. Place a pillow behind your head if your neck is uncomfortable.
- Put your arms down by your side then lift them up to the ceiling and slightly back behind your head, as though reaching for the wall behind you. Then move them back down toward your knees. Repeat 10 times, pausing on the tender areas for at least 10 seconds.
- Variation: Open your arms toward the sides of the room into a T position, then return them over your chest. Repeat 10 times.

Note: Avoid placing tennis balls under your neck.

MEET YOUR FASCIA

Knitted between your muscles, bones, tendons, nerves, blood vessels, and organs is a little-known connective tissue called fascia, from the Latin for "band." These large, continuous sheets of soft tissue are in many ways the facilitators of the body — they make sure that the force of muscle movement doesn't harm the other tissues, while also helping muscles change shape and length during movement. Ideally, your fascia would be smooth and supple, allowing for easy, gliding internal movement. However, when subjected to tension, poor posture, stress, inflammation, old injuries, and lack of use, these tissues become thick and tight. Fascia in this state is frequently where pain originates, and it sets the stage for injury, poor digestion, and a frazzled nervous system — all of which is bad for sleep.

One of the best remedies for keeping your fascia "juicy" is foam rolling. By rolling out your fascia, you're encouraging it to become "unstuck," and to allow those sheets of tissues to once again move smoothly. It's a great way to reverse the effects of a day spent sitting, as well as to release any tension you may be carrying with you into bed.

To get started, look for a medium-density roller with a little texture on its surface, which will help knead the tissues and encourage circulation and lymphatic drainage. The roller should be able to support your weight but also have a little give. Some searching online will reveal plenty of exercises you can do with your roller, from opening your chest, to releasing your neck and shoulders, to targeting your hips. Our friend and foam-roller expert Lauren Roxburgh offers great short videos on her site, as well as her own foam roller that she recommends.

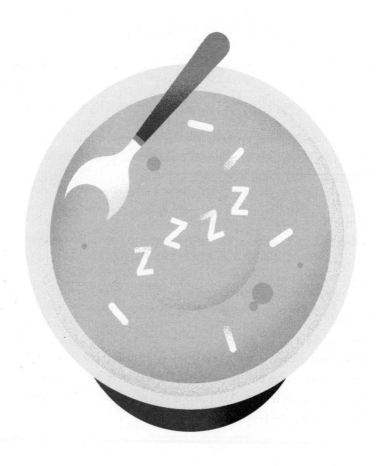

CHAPTER 6

EAT TO SLEEP

You've heard the expression "Live to eat or eat to live," and you can probably guess where this book will land when it comes to that argument. (If you chose "eat to live," then you would be correct). When it comes to sleep, you really are eating to live—healthier, longer, and better. That's because *what* you eat and *when* you eat it has an enormous effect on your rhythm, your sleep, and by extension, your longevity. By "eat" we mean pretty much anything you ingest—food, beverages, alcohol, caffeine, nicotine, medications, herbal medicinals, and natural supplements. Each of these plays a role in either keeping you from deep, restful sleep or nudging your body that much closer to your optimal rhythm. We aren't here to tell you to quit the habits that you enjoy in the name of taking up a monk-like dedication to sleep. All we're asking you to do is get realistic about which behaviors are affecting your night's rest. We can promise that if you do, you're going to feel—and sleep—better.

GET TO THE GUT OF THE MATTER

One of the newest discoveries in sleep research is that there is a link between gut health and sleep. It makes sense: Your entire body—

including your digestive system—is designed to have predictable cycles of sleep, wakefulness, and eating. And by upsetting that rhythm, you throw your entire body off-kilter, gut and all. What we now know is that this is **bi-directional.** Translation: An out-of-rhythm life can create an out-of-rhythm gut, but also an out-of-rhythm gut can create an out-of-rhythm life. Conversely, *good* gut health can create good sleep. The healthier your gut, the easier it is to fall asleep and stay asleep.[50]

So when it comes to giving your sleep wellness a makeover, getting your gut in order is an essential place to start.

Let's break it down further.

Here's What We Know about the Gut:

- **It contains trillions of microorganisms,** mainly bacteria, that live in your gastrointestinal tract. This is called your microbiome. Some of these bacteria are beneficial (health-promoting) and some not so much (inflammation- and disease-promoting). The goal is to keep this constantly shifting balance in favor of the good guys.
- **Everyone's is different.** The health of your microbiome is the result of the microbes you're exposed to in your environment, your diet, and medications you've taken (specifically antibiotics and PPIs).
- **It's also known as your "second brain."** Far from just digesting your food, the gut is also home to a second nervous system, which is constantly communicating with your brain and central nervous system (via the vagus nerve) and influencing hormone production, immune system function, appetite, digestion, metabolism, behavior, mood, and stress responses. This connection is what's called the microbiome-gut-brain axis.
- **It's hormone central.** The gut is the largest endocrine organ in the body and regulates the secretion of neurotransmitters

such as cortisol, tryptophan, and serotonin. In fact, 90 percent of serotonin is made in your gut, not your brain.

- **It's also immune system central.** Seventy percent of the cells that make up your immune system surround your gut, and microbiota interact with these cells to help regulate your immune response.

- **You don't want to piss it off.** Because the microbiome is plugged in to some of the most major systems in your body, an out-of-balance gut is linked to everything from digestive issues like bloating, gas, and constipation to anxiety, depression, and skin conditions like acne and eczema. An imbalanced microbiome can also increase your risk of obesity, diabetes, suppressed immunity, autoimmune disease, and sleep disorders such as insomnia.

- **It's sensitive.** In addition to leading to out-of-rhythm sleep, the balance of your microbiota can be disrupted by diet, stress, illness, and the overuse of medications, in particular antibiotics and PPIs.

So How Does the Gut Affect Sleep?

- Your body's Master Clock works in synergy with your microbiome's clock. If one of these rhythms is disrupted, the other goes too. Jet lag, for example, has been found to disrupt the diversity of gut microbiota, while the microbiome can actually influence the clock gene expression in your suprachiasmatic nucleus (or SCN, home of the Master Clock) and plays a crucial role in maintaining the normal expression of those genes.[51]

- When either the circadian rhythm or microbiome rhythm is upset, it creates a vicious cycle: glucose intolerance, weight gain, and metabolic changes can occur—all of which affect sleep and further distort the overall rhythm.

- Gut bacteria create their own circadian rhythm by calling for the production of cytokines, multipurpose chemical messengers that have a hand in a number of your body's functions, including inducing sleep. Then, when your cortisol levels rise in the morning, cytokine production declines. However, an imbalanced, out-of-rhythm gut won't be able to maintain this cadence.

- The microbiome has the ability to create the same sleep-influencing neurotransmitters as the brain, namely dopamine, serotonin, melatonin, and GABA. But a disordered gut cannot rise to this challenge and create sufficient amounts.

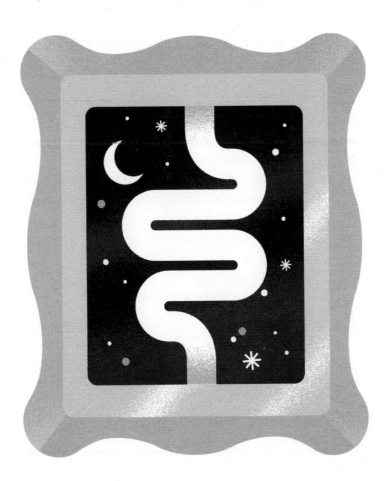

HEAL YOUR MICROBIOME

Your microbiome begins to develop at birth and is affected throughout your life by many (oftentimes surprising) factors. Whether you were born vaginally or via C-section, if you were breastfed, if you smoke, the quality of your diet, the amount of stress you experience, exercise habits, sleep hygiene, and whether you've used antibiotics or other medications can significantly affect the quality and diversity of your microbiome, for better and worse. So while you may have had experiences or made decisions in the past that haven't exactly supported a healthy, balanced microbiome, know that you can begin to change that now.

Your microbiome—like your body—is designed for predictable cycles of sleep, wakefulness, and eating. So as you bring yourself back into rhythm by adopting new habits, your gut will follow suit. But one of the biggest influencers on your microbiome's health is your diet. We highly recommend kicking things off with The Reset (page 225), which is one way to become more mindful about rebalancing and recalibrating your microbiome. Then refer to these simple tips for *keeping* your gut in rhythm. It may be uncomfortable at first, but just remember: You have to take care of your gut for it to take care of you.

The Gut-in-Rhythm Rules to Live By

Pass on sugary, starchy, and processed foods.

We'll explain this in greater detail in just a minute, but if it's sweet or starchy, and especially if it was produced in a food factory, it's not good for you or your microbiome. High-in-sugar foods and easily digested starch like pastries and processed breads mostly get broken down in the small intestine, which can result in the proliferation of harmful bacteria there, leading to SIBO, or small intestinal bacterial overgrowth. Adding insult to injury, processed foods contain nasty stuff like trans fats, preservatives, artificial sweeteners, artificial ingredients, genetically modified organisms (GMOs), and industrial seed oils, all of which can wreak even more havoc on the microbiome—so get them off your plate.

Avoid glyphosate sprayed crops.

Glyphosate is the active ingredient in the highly toxic pesticide known as Roundup, which is used not only to ward off pests on GMO crops but is also used on conventional plants (particularly grains) to chemically expedite the dying process of these crops so they can be dried and harvested more quickly (yum?). In addition, it's a registered antibiotic, making the stuff awful for your body and even worse for gut health. Crops typically sprayed by glyphosate include corn, peas, soybeans, flax, rye, lentils, triticale, buckwheat, canola, millet, potatoes, sugar beets, soybeans, and edible legumes.

You can sidestep the bad stuff by choosing organic at the grocery store or buying from your local farmers market. This will also ensure that you won't be ingesting fertilizers or other types of pesticides, which can be harmful to the beneficial bacteria in your gut and alter your microbiome makeup.

Add prebiotics to your plate.

Prebiotics are food fibers that most of our digestive system can't break down, but the bacteria in our microbiome most certainly can. They're like microflora superfoods, giving your good bacteria the high-octane fuel they need to do all the things that keep your gut healthy, like protecting the gut wall, digesting your food, keeping the bad guys in check, contributing to your immune system, and coordinating with your central nervous system. Foods that are rich in prebiotic fiber include: garlic, onions, radishes, leeks, asparagus, Jerusalem artichokes, dandelion greens, broccoli, chicory root, lentils, and chickpeas.

And don't throw away the tough and stalky bits of your veggies! Those chewier, fibrous bites—especially broccoli and asparagus stalks—are particularly nutritious for gut bacteria. You could also opt to take a prebiotic supplement, making sure that it's a real fiber source and contains one or more of these ingredients: inulin, FOS (fructo-oligosaccharides), pectin, arabinogalactan, chicory root, acacia fiber, artichoke fiber, and green banana fiber.

Get funky with fermented foods.

Fermented foods like sauerkraut, yogurt, kimchi (Korean fermented cabbage), miso, and kefir (fermented milk) come loaded with their own beneficial bacteria that join forces with the good stuff in your gut. The research suggests that the newcomers help the longtime residents do a better job of protecting your health—so add a few servings a week to your plate.

Skip conventionally farmed meat, poultry, dairy products, and eggs.

Conventionally farmed animals such as cows, pigs, and chickens are almost always fed large amounts of antibiotics to prevent them from getting sick and to fatten them up before slaughter. Those antibiotics then end up in you when you consume those products. In addition, many of these animals are given hormones and likely fed GMO corn or soy too. Not exactly the menu your gut was hoping for.

Minimize your antibiotic use.

In Frank's opinion, antibiotics are one of the most overused medications. Sure, every so often a raging infection may warrant antibiotics, but much of the time they're unnecessary and can lead to potentially dangerous antibiotic resistance. Inside the gut, they're indiscriminate killers, taking out the good bacteria along with the bad. Whenever possible, go with herbal "antibiotics" or anti-microbial herbs. They tend to be tougher on the toxic bacteria you want to get rid of and easier on your good bacteria. If your practitioner prescribes them, ask whether there's possible alternative treatments available. Or consider working with a practitioner, such as a functional medicine doctor, who won't rely so heavily on such medications.

Steer clear of the proton-pump inhibitors (PPIs).

There's good research that people who rely on stomach acid blockers (like Nexium, Prilosec, etc.) are less likely to have a diverse collection of bacteria in the gut. That means greater vulnerability to leaky gut and digestive or immunity problems. The primary goal should be to reduce your need for PPIs altogether, which can frequently be accomplished through diet (while simultaneously benefiting other areas of your health as well).

Take advantage of a daily probiotic.

A probiotic is a supplement that provides your gut with more beneficial microorganisms. Although it's always best to get your probiotics from food, you can also enjoy the advantages of fermented foods in easy supplement form, either a capsule or powder. If you are taking an antibiotic, balance it out with a high-quality probiotic to help keep your belly on an even keel.

Filter your water.

Chlorinated water kills harmful bugs and tamps down many waterborne diseases. However, it can also do a number on the good bacteria in your microbiome. To protect your gut from some of the chlorine damage, invest in a good water filter that will leave the chlorine out of your cup.

Mend your mind.

Just as your gut can influence emotions via the gut-brain axis, your gut is also sensitive to the emotion, stress, anxiety, and depression that your brain dishes out. Mood is also a big factor in how well you sleep, which is why many of our "live to sleep" recommendations in Chapter 5 address how to breathe a little deeper and stress a little less. These new habits will do double duty, quieting the mind for a good night's rest while also changing the mental wavelengths that affect your gut health.

Live the lifestyle.

Remember, your gut is a microcosm of your larger body. The habits that are designed to keep you in rhythm and improve your overall health—exercising, embracing consistency in your daily routine, cutting back on drinking, quitting smoking—will ultimately benefit your microbiome too.

CHOOSE SWEET DREAMS OVER SUGAR

We consider ourselves reasonable people. We're nice guys. And we told you that this book is all about picking and choosing habits that work for you. But when it comes to sugar, that all changes. Today is the day you're going to get this sleep-sabotaging, brain-distorting, hormone-skewing, health-bombing crap out of your life.

When it comes to your rhythm, it doesn't get much worse than sugar. Sugary foods and drinks take your hormones for a roller-coaster ride so that you don't register hunger the way you normally should, making you eat more, and more often, and then store those calories as fat. It jacks up your "reward" hormones so that you need bigger and bigger hits of the stuff just to get that nice, tasty high. Sound familiar? It should: sugar is just as addictive as tobacco, alcohol, and even heroin. And speaking of alcohol, sugar in the form of fructose is just as hard on your liver and is converted into fat. When eaten repeatedly—as we're wired to do—sugar sets you up for weight gain, high blood sugar, body-wide inflammation, diabetes, heart disease, cancer, dementia, depression, and infertility.

As for sleep, as though any of the aforementioned conditions weren't enough to disrupt the cycles that your body relies on for getting restorative rest, sugar can also cause a host of other issues:

- A 2016 study confirmed that higher sugar intake is associated with lighter, less restorative sleep and more night wakings.[52] Ever felt the full-body hangover that is a sugar crash? That can happen even when you're sleeping, causing you to wake up.
- Another study from Columbia University concluded that a diet high in refined carbohydrates—particularly added sugars—is linked to a higher risk of insomnia, especially in women aged 50 and over.[53]
- When your blood sugar spikes, your body reacts by releasing insulin, which drops your blood sugar but ultimately leads to the release of adrenaline and cortisol, which—as you may remember—are the hormone equivalents of your morning coffee with an extra shot.
- Metabolizing sugar uses up a lot of magnesium. You need this essential mineral for supporting your levels of GABA, a neurotransmitter that promotes sleep.
- When sugar spikes your pleasure center's dopamine stores, it distorts a crucial rhythm that regulates when the body needs to eat. High-calorie foods (aka those high in sugar as well as fat—not the healthy, unprocessed kind) trick your body into thinking it needs more food, particularly food with more fat

and, you guessed it, more sugar. This sets off a cascade of consequences: It leads you to further saturate your diet with health-disrupting foods, and it also knocks off-kilter the messages your body is getting about what it needs and when.[54] And as you'll see in the next section, when you eat is also a factor in preserving your daily rhythm, not just what you're eating.

Don't Sleep on Hidden Sugars

You've probably heard it before, but we'll say it again: You're most likely eating more sugar than you think. If you're eating any processed food (anything that comes in a package), there's a good chance that manufacturers have hidden some kind of sweetener in there, whether it's for taste, as a cheap preservative, or just to keep you hooked. These tend to be labeled as "added sugars" and include cane sugar and high-fructose corn syrup, but they can also be more misleading in the case of "healthy" or "natural" sweeteners like honey, agave, maple syrup, and fruit juice. But unless a sugar is bound by fiber (like naturally occurring sugars in fruits and vegetables), there's no such thing as healthy or natural. Make sure to check the labels of everything you're eating, especially your condiments, dressings, snack bars, and drinks, where hidden sugars are often lurking.

EAT IN RHYTHM

While light and dark are the primary influencers on your Master Clock, there's another major authority that helps set your rhythm: eating. When you eat your meals is how your secondary clock (your digestive system) figures out what time of day it is and sets its own 24-hour cycle. It does this mainly so it can calibrate when to release digestive enzymes, absorb nutrients, send out the waste, and tend to repairs. Your microbiome also has its own circadian rhythm, which it uses to adjust the balance of specialized bacteria it has on hand— some bacteria are more numerous during daylight hours, and others at night.

Thanks to the gut-brain instant messaging system, your gut is constantly coordinating with the Master Clock in your brain to give it reports about what's happening in its neighborhood. But if your Master Clock is on a different page, then your overall rhythm suffers. So even though you might be getting enough sleep, your gut could be pulling your whole tempo off beat. The result is essentially jet lag, resulting in symptoms like brain fog, fatigue, digestive issues, imbalance in your microbiome, and—over time—more serious chronic conditions.

One of the most effective ways to return to your gut's optimal cycle is to eat in rhythm with the day. You want to think of your meals as a way to get back to your body's preprogrammed factory settings, because your body is naturally equipped to receive specific amounts of food at specific times.

Here's a look at your digestive tract's circadian rhythm (which your microbiome's rhythm is attuned to and a big fan of):

6 a.m. to 10 a.m. The digestive furnace starts to boot up for the day. It's not at full blast just yet, but it's looking for kindling to build the fire.

10 a.m. to 2 p.m. Your metabolism is at its full, fiery peak, ready to incinerate food into sustenance and energy that the whole body can use. Your insulin sensitivity is highest now, meaning your body is equipped to harness any glucose you take in as fuel.

2 p.m. to 6 p.m. Your digestion's pilot light progressively wanes until the evening, as does your insulin sensitivity.

6 p.m. to 10 p.m. Your body begins to shift into a slower, quieter mode, getting ready to power down for sleep.

10 p.m. to 2 a.m. Your digestive furnace fires up again, but not to work on the bowl of Lucky Charms you snuck in before bed. This rekindling is meant to take place while you're asleep, so that the digestive system can tend to repairs and other maintenance activities—which it can only do if digestion of your food is complete. This is why when you stay up later than 10 p.m. you tend to feel like you've gotten a second wind, and also why your appetite revs up late at night. Those midnight munchies are not true hunger pangs; they're just your digestion working overtime to take out the trash.

The Eat-to-Sleep Meal Planner

In order to fully re-sync your sleep rhythm, you have to change your eating patterns to support your body's digestive cycle. Consider this your new menu for sleep:

- *Choose consistent mealtimes.* Like your puppy, your body learns to anticipate feeding time, releasing enzymes and hormones to help you digest. Eating at the same time every day not only ensures that you're digesting properly, but it also guarantees that the ebb and flow of your metabolism will be in sync with your Master Clock. This goes for the weekends too. By changing up your habit rhythm just those two days a week, you're inflicting social jet lag on your rhythm. And suffice it to say that your body's natural functions don't observe the days of the week.

■ *Break the fast gently.* The morning is when your body is shifting back into day mode, but hasn't fully hit its stride. Gently introduce food to your digestive system with a light, nutrient-rich breakfast. Smoothies are a particularly great way to deliver maximum nutrition without a lot of stress on digestion. Another sleep-promoting breakfast option is to not eat a morning meal and follow an intermittent fasting protocol, which we'll talk more about on page 141.

■ *Eat your biggest meal midday.* Your digestive system is primed to receive the majority of its fuel in the middle of the day, between 10 a.m. and 2 p.m. Feed your system with a robust (ideally whole-food, veggie-filled) brunch or lunch that delivers most of your daily nourishment. This will alleviate how much you feel the need to eat in the evening, when your digestive flame begins to dim.

■ *Redefine dinner.* Eating a large meal in the evening is a relatively new idea and one that we've attached a lot of sentimentality to. Yes, it's a nice time to socialize and reflect on the day—and those things don't have to change—but eating a lot of food late in the day is not doing your digestion—or your waistline—any favors. By the time the sun starts to set, your digestive tract is preparing for its nighttime shift. So the later in the day you eat, the higher the chance that your food won't be properly digested, leading to things like acid reflux, cramping, and digestive upset. It's also making your digestive system work overtime, giving you less restful sleep and skewing the balance of microflora that usually inhabit the gut at nighttime (setting you up for more bad sleep). Also, when you routinely eat your biggest meal at night, you are prompting your body to produce ghrelin, the hunger hormone, when production would normally be waning for the day. This ultimately trains your body to get hungry when it wouldn't normally be and interrupts an important hormonal rhythm, while also causing your body to store abdominal fat.

Your body actually prefers to be fasted for sleep so it can prioritize recovery and rebuilding during sleep instead of working on your dinner. So bottom line: Eat a light evening meal, at least two to three hours before you go to bed. Even better, go for four. And if you do eat late one night, don't stay up trying to hit the two-hour mark. Just go to bed and start fresh the next day.

GIVE YOUR DIGESTION A REST: OVERNIGHT FASTING

Brief, periodic fasts are the norm for humans—it wasn't exactly like we had food on-demand back in the day. And we now know that intentionally observing a short period without eating, also known as intermittent fasting, is beneficial for a number of reasons:

- Your digestive system is more resilient when it doesn't have to be digesting your food all the time.
- It helps your metabolism and hormones re-sync their 24-hour cycle.
- It tells your metabolism to burn fat that is stored on the body.
- It allows your body to experience a longer-than-normal period of low insulin in the blood, which tells your body to burn energy to keep insulin low (the opposite of what happens when you're eating a continuous stream of food).
- It's a great example of hormesis, or a way to gently stress your body in order to stimulate its detoxifying, renewing, and repairing energies.
- It activates autophagy, a body-wide cellular repair process that removes waste material from cells and quells inflammation, slows aging, and optimizes mitochondria function, giving you greater protection against disease and helping you feel and look better.

But most importantly, by fasting overnight—and hitting the ideal 16-hour mark between meals—you're helping to put your eating back in rhythm. You're delaying your first meal until your digestion and metabolism are at their strongest, and you're encouraged to eat an earlier dinner, and less of it. By the time you have your last meal of the day, get a good night's rest, and wake up, you've essentially already fasted—done and done. And you're letting your body do its thing at night, giving you deeper, better rest and making your Master Clock and all its minion clocks very, very happy.

Essentially, overnight fasting is a lot like good sleep. The therapeutic benefits are body-wide and lead to positive downstream shifts like weight loss, metabolic regulation, stable blood sugar, decreased blood pressure, and looking and feeling younger.

There're a lot of fasting protocols out there (also called "intermittent fasting" or "time-restricted eating"), so we're keeping things simple:

- Simply wait about 16 hours between your last meal of Day 1 and your first meal of Day 2. If you finish dinner at 8 p.m., you'll "break the fast" around 12 p.m. the following day. If you have dinner at 6 p.m., your next meal will be around 10 a.m. (Studies show that 16 hours is when autophagy, the body's self-cleaning mechanism, kicks in.)
- If you need to, build up over time. Start with 12 hours (the ideal for good digestion and overnight detoxification) and build up from there. Remember, you're sleeping for 8 of those hours!
- Do it one to two times a week for basic preventive measures. Do it every day for a gold star. Do what works for you; it doesn't have to be all or nothing.
- Don't worry about exercising in the morning on an empty stomach. But working out after you wake up can be beneficial, prompting your body to burn stored fat for energy instead of the glucose from your food.
- Drink water. Or, as a second-best option, tea. Third best would be black coffee—and if you really must, add a bit of pure fat, like MCT (medium-chain triglycerides) oil, cream, or

unsweetened milk alternatives, which won't trigger insulin production the way sugar or milk will. Water is ideal because anything else will call your liver into action and can put an end to autophagy. But there is a counterargument that so long as you don't trigger an insulin response (which is something carbohydrates would do), then you're still technically fasting.

- Stop it already with the sugar. Quitting sugary foods will make fasting easier. Many people find that omitting all grains and sometimes legumes from their diet also helps. That's why The Reset (page 225) is a great time to introduce overnight fasting.
- Skip all of the above if you are pregnant, nursing, on multiple medications, an athlete with rigorous training, underweight (BMI<18.5), or under the age of 18. Also, if you would describe yourself as "extremely stressed" or feel emotionally distraught, cool it with the (albeit short-lived) hormesis—your body doesn't need the extra burden right now. As always, feel free to consult your doctor if you have any concerns.

TRY A SOBER SLUMBER

We, and a lot of scientists, can authoritatively say it: Alcohol is terrible for sleep. It might feel like that glass of wine is helping you get nice and drowsy, but even one alcoholic drink in the evening can disrupt your sleep cycle. Booze causes you to wake multiple times in the night (often imperceptibly, except for the extra times you have to pee), and it keeps you from entering the deeper stages of sleep, which throws a big wrench in many of your body's restorative practices. On top of that, you end up waking up still feeling tired, despite maybe having spent a respectable amount of time in bed. That then leads to a choose-your-own-adventure of consequences from not being properly rested: craving sugar and carbs for a quick hit of energy, being too tired to exercise, and compensating with caffeine—all of which messes up your next night's sleep and the cycle continues.

The Conclusion

The more you drink, and the closer your drinking is to bedtime, the more it will negatively affect your sleep. Even two drinks a day is enough to create a sleep disturbance that extends beyond the 24-hour cycle in which you were drinking.

Our Recommendations

Consider real life, but be a grown-up about it.

We get that a drink is a nice way to celebrate with friends or wash down a meal, or maybe it's even part of your job. We just ask that you consider the effect that it may be having on your sleep and then make the mature choice for you. After The Reset (page 225), which calls for no alcohol, you may find that you don't miss it. Or at least you'll have a baseline for experimenting with whether or not alcohol is an issue for your sleep.

Consider the time of day when you're drinking.

Studies have shown that the body can more effectively process alcohol, like food, at certain times of the day than others.[55] It turns out your body is attuned to Happy Hour, metabolizing alcohol best in the early to middle-evening hours. And it is least equipped to handle alcohol in the morning, which pretty much any person after a three-mimosa brunch could tell you.

And consider the type of alcohol.

Go with a low-carb, low-sugar option, if possible. High-quality tequila (without the sugary mixers), when made from 100 percent agave, tends to not have the same hangover-y effect as other liquors. Vodka and gin are good options too. But we think the best, cleanest, pro-sleep buzz is going to be from something a little more herbal. (See "Go Green," page 158, and "Take a [Natural] Chill Pill," page 169).

Sleeping Under the Influence

Despite its popular use as a sleep aid—it's estimated that 20 percent of people rely on alcohol in some form as a pre-bed assist—alcohol essentially keeps you up all night in a number of ways:

- Primarily, alcohol shifts your sleep homeostasis, which is how your body manages your need for sleep according to how long you've been awake. To do this, your body uses adenosine, a chemical produced in the brain. The longer you're awake, the more adenosine accumulates. And the more adenosine accumulates, the more it can block other chemicals that stimulate wakefulness, and the more "sleep pressure" builds, which is our biological urge to sleep that naturally increases as the day wears on. Alcohol artificially elevates your levels of adenosine, overriding your body's natural buildup. This prematurely releases the sleep pressure release valve and throws off your natural sleep-wake cycle.
- As alcohol is metabolized by the liver, its sedative effects dissipate, and the body goes through what's called a "rebound effect." This includes a shift from deeper to lighter sleep, including more awakenings and ultimately less time spent in slow-wave sleep and, potentially, REM.
- Alcohol suppresses melatonin production, which as you know is essential for your body to keep day and

night straight. Research indicates that even a moderate dose of alcohol up to an hour before bedtime can reduce melatonin production by nearly 20 percent.[56]

- Wine, beer, and sugary mixers are high in carbohydrates and turn to sugar in the body. When your blood sugar crashes in the middle of the night, it causes a stress response in the body, which disrupts your sleep.
- Drinking before bed induces slow-wave sleep patterns, or delta activity. That's a good thing for sleep. But it also turns on alpha activity, which is more of the wavelength you're on when resting quietly, but awake. These two settings are at odds with each other and ultimately inhibit restorative sleep.
- Alcohol causes the whole body to relax, including your throat muscles, which aggravates breathing problems like snoring and sleep apnea.
- People who drink alcohol—even a small amount—late in the evening, are potentially less likely to respond to important light cues in the morning, which further upsets the Master Clock.[57]

CURB CAFFEINE

We get it—you're tired, dragging, fuzzy in the head, and need a boost. What could be more inviting than caffeine, one of the most perfect drugs nature has ever created? It gives you an almost instant second (or third or fourth) wind, laser-focuses your mind, and potentially helps you burn more calories at the gym. But when it comes to sleep? Total buzzkill. This was one of Neil's biggest hurdles—he loved drinking coffee. But doing it all day made a mess of his rhythm.

That's because caffeine is a stimulant, and the way it revs you up is by blocking the receptors in your brain that recognize the sleep-inducing neurotransmitter adenosine. Adenosine is what builds up in your system as you accumulate waking hours, creating sleep pressure or the urge to sleep. Caffeine basically stops that from happening, tricking the brain into believing it's not tired. But the longer caffeine blocks adenosine, the more of it builds up in your system. When the effects of caffeine eventually wear off, all that backlogged adenosine comes rushing back into the brain, making you feel even more tired than before you had that cup of coffee/black tea/energy drink. (They don't call it crashing for nothing.) Plus, caffeine also inhibits melatonin production, even more so than bright light. So now you need caffeine to wake up and function, which makes you sleepier, which causes you to need more caffeine—aka the "caffeine causality loop."

If you want to help your sleep, you need to catch that loop mid-stream and reset the rhythm. The way to do that is to be smarter about how much caffeine you're having and when you're having it:

- **Have a caffeine cap.** We recommend having your last hit of caffeine no later than 1 p.m. Caffeine has a half-life of roughly

five to seven hours, meaning that five to seven hours after
you drink a cup of coffee, half the caffeine is still in your body.
If you're a slow metabolizer (see below), it could take even
longer.

- **Try cutting back.** There's a difference between that 200-
milligram 20-ounce latte and a 50-milligram shot of espresso
in terms of how long it takes the body to break down all that
caffeine. For Neil, a great solution was switching to half-caf
Americanos because he still got to feel like he was drinking
coffee all day, but at only 45 to 75 mg of caffeine a pop (because
it's just one shot of caffeine and one shot of decaf). Even three to
four half-caf Americanos a day would come to around 150 mg
total, versus the 500 to 600 mg of full-strength. We
recommend keeping your total daily intake to 400 milligrams
or less, the equivalent of four 8-ounce cups of coffee. However,
if you determine that you are a slow metabolizer, you may
want to reduce that number. You could also look for an
alternative source, like L-theanine, an amino acid that can
increase focus when taken as a supplement or consumed in
green tea.

- **Be mindful of hidden caffeine.** Caffeine pops up in all kinds
of places, especially chocolate and certain medications. These
sources count toward your total daily tally.

- **Be honest with yourself.** If you feel awful after you drink
caffeine — most likely because you're a slow metabolizer — then
ask yourself why you're reaching for it in the first place,
especially if it's affecting your sleep at night. You'll find that as
you follow your sleep-better protocol, you'll feel less and less of
a need for the caffeine crutch.

WHAT'S YOUR CAFFEINE METABOLISM TYPE?

New research into how we process caffeine has unearthed that there are two kinds of people: Those who metabolize caffeine quickly (and can have a shot of espresso before bed with no issue falling asleep), and those who are slow metabolizers (the ones who drink a cup of coffee in the morning and feel anxious and jittery all day). This depends on which "caffeine gene" you carry:

CYP1A2 codes for an enzyme that helps break down caffeine and contributes to its faster metabolization.

CYP1A2 *1F is a mutation of CYP1A2 and does pretty much the opposite, resulting in the slower metabolism of caffeine.

Genome testing (like that offered by 23andMe, 3x4 Genetics, Genelex, and Gene Planet) can tell you which camp you fall into, but you can also pretty accurately figure it out through self-diagnosis: Ask yourself how you feel physically, mentally, and emotionally a few hours after you have caffeine. Slow metabolizers tend to feel sort of strung-out afterward (sometimes for up to nine hours!) while their speedier counterparts merely feel more energetic and alert.

STOP SMOKING ALREADY

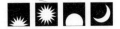

Let's just cut to the chase: In addition to all the terrible things that smoking causes (emphysema, chronic bronchitis, asthma, heart disease, heart attack, stroke, premature aging, oral cancer, lung cancer, and kidney cancer, in addition to making you smell like an ashtray), it is also actively working against your sleep. Nicotine—which is found in both cigarettes and vaping cartridges—is a stimulant with effects linked to deep-sleep suppression. Research shows that smokers spend more time sleeping lightly than nonsmokers, costing them the benefits of slow-wave sleep. So save the deep inhalations for chilling out instead.

Nicotine withdrawal is also linked to lowered quality of sleep, but it's a temporary setback that the rest of your sleep-better protocol will compensate for before long.

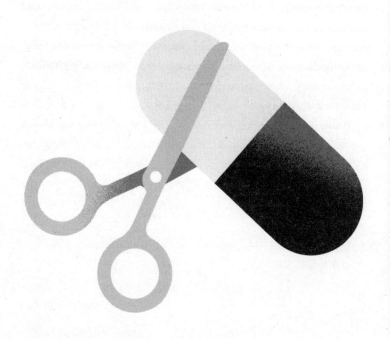

EDIT YOUR MEDS

Getting a better night's rest could be as simple as reducing or omitting the dosage of your prescription and over-the-counter medications. Many pharmaceuticals interfere with sleep as a side effect, directly and indirectly. For example, medications for high blood pressure and asthma can cause insomnia, while some cold, cough, and flu medications upset your sleep-wake cycle by inducing drowsiness. Meanwhile, many medications like PPIs, antibiotics, and SSRIs stress your gut, unbalance your microbiome, disrupt your hormones, and increase inflammation[58]—all of which causes downstream sleep issues.

When you take a medication, it's not doing nothing. And it's not working in a vacuum, only targeting what you're taking it for. Rather, it's changing your entire inner landscape, interrupting or turning off certain natural processes. As a result, you experience side effects, anything from weight gain and mood swings, to headaches and digestive issues, to abnormal heart rhythms and increased blood pressure. All of these effects disrupt your health, throw off your natural rhythms, and affect your sleep. In fact, a study published in a prominent medical journal found that almost 65 percent of side effects found in drug trials are left out of the reports that doctors use to make treatment decisions.

We're not anti-meds. But we are anti–not getting to the root of your health issues. And when it comes to many medications, they're usually prescribed to merely treat the *symptoms* you're experiencing, not the underlying issue itself. Yes, some medications can be lifesaving in critical situations, but for the most part, many of the pharmaceuticals that people are given can cause more harm than good. And a great deal of research shows that in many cases diet, supplements, stress relief, and improved sleep work better than any medication ever could.

This goes back to what we put forth in the Introduction of this book: If the leaves of a tree start turning yellow, you don't just paint them green. You don't just manage the symptoms and call it a cure. Instead, you get to the root of the problem to see what's causing those leaves to turn yellow. The same goes for your sleep-better protocol—poor sleep is a symptom of underlying issues that need to be addressed, in addition to sometimes being the root issue that's causing other symptoms to arise. Either way, the solution isn't to take three Ambien and call it a day. No, it's reevaluating your diet, lifestyle, and environment in order to bring your entire rhythm back in sync. The same goes for addressing the health issues you're treating with medication. And as luck would have it, many of these conditions can be successfully mitigated through diet, lifestyle, environment, and—you guessed it—better sleep.

MEDICATIONS THAT ARE NOTORIOUS SLEEP DISRUPTORS

- Antiarrhythmics (for heart rhythm problems)
- Beta blockers (for high blood pressure)
- Clonidine (for high blood pressure)
- Corticosteroids (for inflammation or asthma)
- Diuretics (for high blood pressure)
- Cough, cold, and flu medications that contain alcohol
- Headache and pain medications that contain caffeine
- Nicotine replacement products
- Sedating antihistamines (for colds and allergies)
- SSRIs (for depression or anxiety)
- Sympathomimetic stimulants (for attention deficit disorder)
- Theophylline (for asthma)
- Thyroid hormone (for hypothyroidism)[59]

Writing Your Sleep Rx

- Do some research about the root causes of the conditions you're affected by. Read about existing alternative treatments for these issues — that can be used in tandem with medication or instead of it — so that you can develop a strategy from an informed, empowered place.
- Never stop taking a medication on your own. Instead, do an inventory of all the medications you are currently taking, and ask your health care provider:
  - What does this medication do?
  - Is this drug intended to cure my underlying condition?
  - What are the potential negative side effects?
  - What is the evidence that this drug is actually effective?
  - Are there natural alternatives I might try first?
- Find an advocate. If your doctor isn't willing to explore alternative treatment methods with you, you may want to seek out one who does. Functional medicine doctors are trained to search for root causes in their patients and often reach for diet and lifestyle changes before prescription medication, working with you and your budget to create a protocol that fits. To find a practitioner near you, check out functionalmedicine.org.

WHEN DIET, EXERCISE, STRESS RELIEF, ALTERNATIVE MEDICINE, AND SUPPLEMENTS MIGHT WORK BETTER THAN DRUGS

Moderately high blood pressure (a systolic reading consistently between 140 and 160)

Coronary artery disease

Moderately high blood sugar and early-stage Type 2 diabetes

Arthritis

Aches and pains

Viral upper respiratory infections

Colds and sinusitis

Prevention and treatment of migraine and chronic headache

Heartburn and acid reflux (gastroesophageal reflux disease — GERD)

Irritable bowel syndrome (IBS)

Acne, psoriasis, eczema, and many other skin conditions

Mild and moderate depression

Mild and moderate anxiety

Many autoimmune diseases

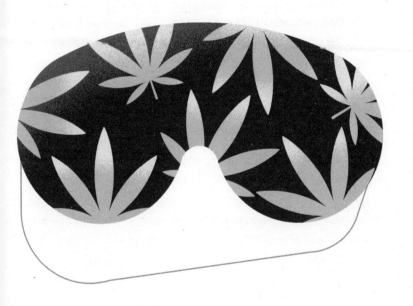

GO GREEN

Partaking in legally available cannabis products such as CBD is a big trend—although it's less about getting high and more about getting well. There's now growing scientific evidence that the benefits of this plant—which many ancient healing traditions have long recognized—extend way beyond its recreational use, especially when it comes to sleep. We like to think of it as the "anti-drug" of choice—it's an anti-inflammatory, antibacterial, antispasmodic, antioxidant, anticonvulsant, antidepressant, antipsychotic, antitumoral, and antianxiety. Not to mention the fact that it comes with none of the common potential risks—from toxic ingredients to side effects to likelihood of overdose or physical addiction—that its pharmaceutical counterparts do. The medical establishment now recognizes that some active compounds in cannabis (most notably cannabidiol, aka CBD) can alleviate things like insomnia, stress, anxiety, and inflammation. And in Frank's practice, CBD is one of the most common "prescriptions" he gives to his patients for sleep, namely because it's calming, safe, effective, and natural. Consider it a very worthwhile addition to your plant-medicine cabinet.

What Is CBD?

CBD is one of over 100 compounds, known as cannabinoids, found in the marijuana plant. Unlike another prevalent compound in marijuana, THC or tetrahydrocannabinol, CBD doesn't cause psychoactive effects or change one's state of mind. What CBD does appear to do, however, is stimulate our endocannabinoid system. This in-house feel-good factory regulates our body's internal balance, encourages the body to heal, elevates our mood, modulates anxiety and fear, strengthens immunity, fosters fertility and reproductive health, and helps us endure stress. While we make our own endocannabinoids (responsible for such things as a "runner's high"), we further stimulate and strengthen this system when we bring in outside sources like CBD or THC.

What's the Difference between CBD and THC?

Simply put, THC gets you high, while CBD does not. CBD works indirectly with your endocannabinoid system, while THC works more directly. While both compounds have their merits, CBD and THC do best as a team, working together to boost their respective curative powers. For example, CBD can enhance THC's painkilling and anticancer abilities, while taming its mind-altering qualities. CBD keeps THC highs on the lower end of the spectrum, enabling patients to have a longer-lasting, relaxing, yet non-intoxicating experience.

Even though THC has a lot of therapeutic benefits—including relieving underlying stress and anxiety that may make sleep difficult—its psychoactive side effects make it less useful for daily life, and there is some clinical evidence that it can reduce REM sleep. CBD, on the other hand, can be an ideal daily treatment.

What Should I Look for in a CBD Product?

There are thousands of CBD products on the market now, and their quality and concentration can vary widely. That's why buying from reputable sources is always the preferred route. Some of the brands we like are Charlotte's Web, the Alchemist's Kitchen, Lord Jones, and Flora + Bast. Otherwise, we suggest looking for manufacturers who:

- source their products from organic plants or those that contain as few pesticides and chemicals as possible
- extract the oil using solvent-free processes

- submit their products for third-party testing and publish the results

Also, remember that CBD and THC work best together, so THC will also be present in most CBD products in small, legal proportions. This will help boost medicinal effects without inducing a high, though some feeling of increased relaxation may be a pleasant side effect.

How Do I Take CBD?

Forms

Oils and tinctures: Under-the-tongue drops get CBD straight into the bloodstream, though you may not feel the effects for 30 to 90 minutes.

Sprays: These are similar to tinctures, and are taken sublingually.

Capsules and softgels: These are great for beginners because they offer a consistent, straightforward dosage, though they are a slower method of delivery.

Gummies/edibles: They're delicious, but the slowest delivery system (and often contain other additives like sugar).

Patches: They're typically a more concentrated form of CBD and are ideal for extended-release CBD that goes directly into the bloodstream.

Salves and ointments: Topical applications are most effective for localized discomfort, like joint pain and muscle aches.

Smoke/vape: This is the quickest delivery method, but know that vape products are inconsistent in their quality, with some containing less-than-healthful additives.

Dosage

Frank's sleep-solution dosage is 40 to 160 mg CBD per day. That said, how much CBD is ideal for you will depend on your body type, your tolerance, and the concentration of a product. You may need to experiment a bit to learn your ideal dosage, but know that there is a very low risk with overdoing it—you'd need to ingest almost 20,000 mg of CBD oil in a short amount of time in order for it to be toxic to your system—and even then, you still wouldn't experience the mind-altering consequences of taking in too much THC. Start on the low end of the dosage recommendation for a few days and slowly increase until you get the desired results. If you experience things like agitation, diarrhea, or nausea, that is an indication that the dose is too high for you.

Does CBD Have Any Potential Drug Interactions and Side Effects?

Many small-scale studies have found CBD to be safe and well-tolerated at a range of doses. But if you're on a regular regimen of prescription or over-the-counter meds, it's best to clear CBD with your doctor first, as CBD products can interfere with your body's ability to metabolize some medications.

When it comes to CBD's side effects, they are minimal and manageable, with some reports of minor fatigue, changes in weight or appetite, and/or diarrhea. For most of those who use it, regardless of dose, CBD has no significant impact on the central nervous system, vital signs, or mood.

BRIGHTEN UP YOUR VITAMIN D

Vitamin D—that crucial micronutrient that we get from the sun—is so important to our overall health that it's almost mind-boggling how often it's overlooked by traditional doctors. Numerous studies have shown that a vitamin D deficiency plays a role in almost every major chronic issue, including infertility, PMS, depression, seasonal affective disorder, high blood pressure, diabetes, a dysregulated immune response and autoimmune diseases, Parkinson's, multiple sclerosis, Alzheimer's, and cancer. And we know that it's also linked to a host of sleep issues, including sleep disruption, insomnia, and overall poor sleep quality.[60]

We highly recommend that you educate yourself about vitamin D, get tested (or test yourself), and then work with your doc to develop a plan to get your levels up to where they should be. Your sleep (and health) depend on it!

So What's the Big D Deal?

Vitamin D is what many call the sunshine vitamin, but it's actually a steroid with hormone-like activities that regulate the functions of over 200 genes and is essential for our growth, development, and ongoing health. A small amount of it comes from the food we eat, and our bodies are able to synthesize some of it from sunshine. But millions of us are falling short, particularly those of us who spend most of our days indoors and out of the sun. And though it might not seem like a big deal, vitamin D deficiency is considered by many experts to be an under-the-radar epidemic that's laying the groundwork for numerous serious diseases. Because vitamin D is involved in supporting essential functions like immunity and cancer prevention, as well as neurological, cardiovascular, and bone health, it's easy to see just how dangerous falling short can be.

Roughly 40 to 75 Percent of Us Are Vitamin D Deficient

An estimated 1 billion people on the planet are vitamin D deficient, and many can be found in the northern parts of the United States. These include:

- **People with indoor lifestyles,** or those who spend most of their time indoors with little exposure to sunlight.
- **Northern souls,** or those who live in the Northern Hemisphere.
- **Darker-skinned people** are frequently vitamin D deficient, because they need more sun to get the same amount of vitamin D as fair-skinned people.
- **Cover-uppers,** or those who keep skin "protected" with clothes head to toe, or slather themselves in sunscreen, preventing the sunlight exposure needed for the skin to synthesize and produce vitamin D.
- **Older folks** have thinner skin and reduced ability to produce vitamin D, so the 50-plus set is more vulnerable to deficiency.
- **Overweight/obese people and those with excess body fat.**
- **Those with gut problems,** whose microbiomes may not be able to absorb enough vitamin D.
- **Pregnant women,** whose vitamin D needs are greater.

Put Yourself to the Test

Buying a vitamin D kit online is an inexpensive way to test your levels and you can use the results as a guide for you and your doctor to develop a plan that's appropriate for your situation. Another reason to work with your doc rather than monitoring levels on your own is to help guard against possible interactions with meds such as cholesterol-lowering drugs, corticosteroids, and seizure medications.

Know What the Results Mean

Remind your doc that you are looking to achieve *optimal* levels, not just borderline okay ones. Most general practitioners look for an "adequate" reading of a serum 25-OH vitamin D level greater than 20 ng/ml, but Frank, and most of his integrative colleagues, know this number is on the low end. So what are the numbers to shoot for? An optimal range of 50 to 80 ng/ml is where you want to be.

D-ficient No More: Your Simple Solution

If moving closer to the equator isn't in the cards, here's what you can do to keep track of your vitamin D level, get it where it needs to be, and support your health no matter where you live:

- **Check your level** twice a year, preferably spring and fall.
- **Expose your skin to the sun**—responsibly, of course. Even 15 minutes a day at midday without sunscreen can help boost levels, depending on your skin tone. To help you monitor sun exposure, pick up a SunFriend device or try an app to help keep on a healthy track.
- **If sun exposure is not an option, make sure you supplement.** There are two choices: Vitamin D3 (cholecalciferol), which is the type of vitamin D your body produces in response to sun exposure, and vitamin D2 (ergocalciferol), which is a synthetic form. Take vitamin D3 and steer clear of vitamin D2.

- Take a vitamin D3 supplement (preferably combined with vitamin K2) with a meal that includes some healthy fat. This is because vitamin D is a fat-soluble vitamin, which means you need to have some fat with it for it to be absorbed. In Frank's experience, most people need anywhere between 2,000 and 10,000 units/day, depending on their blood levels.
- **Be on the lookout** for symptoms like a metallic taste in the mouth, increased thirst, itchy skin, muscle aches and pains, urinary frequency, nausea, diarrhea and/or constipation—all of which can be signs that your D3 dose may be too high, which is very rare.

MELATONIN: MAKE IT, DON'T FAKE IT

There's a big myth—many of Frank's patients, and millions of others, have bought into it—that popping a melatonin pill is a harmless and effective way to get better sleep. The issue with this is that melatonin is a *hormone,* not a vitamin or a magical sleep aid. Like any other hormone therapy (estrogen, testosterone), when you take a melatonin supplement, you're introducing an active biochemical into your body to create physiological shifts. In fact, the United States and Canada are the only two places in the world where you can buy melatonin as an over-the-counter supplement. Everywhere else it's prescription-only. So here in the States, it's not regulated the same way a pharmaceutical medication would be in terms of consistent quality and dosing.

One big issue with taking synthetic melatonin is that melatonin doesn't just push a button in your body to make you sleepy. Rather, it's a chemical signal for your body to start switching off for the day, setting off a cascade of physiological events and metabolic functions. When you introduce additional melatonin into the body, more than just your sleep mechanisms are affected by it. Those effects can extend to things like your digestion and your mood.

But perhaps the biggest problem with taking this hormone in synthetic form is that it can mess with your body's natural melatonin processes. Research has shown that taking melatonin at the wrong time or taking too-large doses can desensitize your melatonin receptors, which can start shutting down your body's ability to use melatonin at all. If you've taken a melatonin supplement, you may have seen this in action, as you need larger and larger doses over time in order for it to feel effective.

Supplementing melatonin is also most likely not solving your underlying sleep issues. If your not-sleeping type is anxiety-, stress-, or gut-related, melatonin won't help that. And it can't make up for any of the other sleep-disrupting habits you may have picked up.

While we prefer the artisanal, locally grown melatonin our bodies have been programmed to make versus a chemical isolate from a science lab, we do recognize that there are some ways that targeted, short-term use of a melatonin supplement can be helpful.

A melatonin supplement could be right for you if:

You have a chronic sleep-rhythm issue. Think of a melatonin supplement as training wheels—a way to temporarily introduce melatonin at the correct time of evening until you can get into a consistent sleep rhythm. You can safely take melatonin for at least one year, but Frank recommends taking it for one month as you prioritize getting into a consistent rhythm, then weaning off over two weeks.

You're older and experience insomnia. With age, we sometimes experience a decline in our endogenous (in-house) melatonin production. A supplement, along with new sleep- and hormone-encouraging habits, can give your system a jump-start.

You need a re-syncing because of a time zone change or daylight-savings time. A melatonin supplement can be helpful in reestablishing a normal sleep pattern if it's been temporarily disrupted. Neil and Frank use supplements strategically for reacclimating when they're traveling.

A Safer Supplement

Dosage: The standard 3 to 5 mg dose often used in the United States is much more than we need for sleep. More is not better and could theoretically inhibit your endogenous melatonin production. We recommend 0.5 to 1 mg of melatonin and taking it on its own, not as part of a blend. Look for a formula that's slow-release (see Timing below).

Product quality: In North America, where melatonin supplements are not regulated, product quality is a concern. Seek out a reliable brand like Pure Encapsulations or Naturemade.

Timing: When taking a melatonin supplement, timing is crucial, and most people get it wrong. Melatonin has a short half-life (about 30 to 45 minutes), so taking a standard-release tablet around bedtime results in a peak too early in the night. Instead, in order to regulate your circadian rhythm, you want to replicate when your body would naturally release melatonin. Normally, natural melatonin levels are low early in the evening, rise steadily through the night, and peak in the last third of sleep. That's why we recommend taking a time-release pill around bedtime or a sublingual regular-release pill in the middle of the night.

Contraindications: Because you're introducing an active hormone into your body, you want to be mindful of how that may affect your health, especially if you're managing a chronic disease. For example, the Arthritis Foundation advises against melatonin for patients with autoimmune disease because it can stimulate the release of proinflammatory cytokines. We recommend consulting your doctor before taking a melatonin supplement.

TAKE A (NATURAL) CHILL PILL

While we're not fans (to say the least) of prescription and over-the-counter sleep aids, we do believe that there are some effective, natural alternatives that can make your transition back into rhythm a little easier. Just like a pill is never going to be the one solution to any of your health woes, these supplements aren't meant to be your one cure-all. But they will support your other sleep-better efforts. Because many of these supplements have a calming effect on the nervous system, they also have the trickle-down benefit of helping with your underlying sleep issues, such as anxiety or stress. The key to figuring out which of these is right for you is personal experimentation—try them one at a time and see which works. Even better, use them in conjunction with your sleep tracking to see if you can isolate whether a certain supplement is helping you get better sleep.

Magnesium

Many people happen to be deficient in this calming mineral, namely because stress depletes our magnesium stores. Frank is a big fan of recommending magnesium to his patients because it's not only key for many functions in the body, it also helps calm the nervous system. There are a few different types of magnesium supplements. Ideally, you'd find a supplement with magnesium L-threonate, which is one of the most absorbable forms of the mineral and can cross the blood-brain barrier. Buffered magnesium and magnesium glycinate are also acceptable forms; magnesium citrate or oxide is ideal if you're also constipated because it's a double-whammy of a relaxant and a laxative. Magnesium usually comes in a pill or powder form, but it's also available as topical lotions. We're also fans of adding some Epsom salts to your baths ("Take a Warm Bath," page 87) because it is a form of magnesium that can be absorbed through the skin.

Recommended dosage: 300 to 500 mg at night

L-theanine

This amino acid, found in tea, is like nature's valium, calming down the nervous system. You can often find this in a blend with other sleep-promoting compounds like GABA, skullcap, passionflower, and magnolia.

Recommended dosage: 100 to 200 mg at night

B Vitamins

B1, B2, B3, B6, and B12 all contribute to maintaining a healthy nervous system, which in turn helps mitigate the effects of stress on the body. Stress can also deplete the amount of B vitamins we have available, which is why supplementing is not a bad idea. Look for a methylated B vitamin with folate.

Recommended dosage: Follow manufacturer's instructions.

Glycine

Another amino acid that we make naturally, glycine plays an essential role in the nervous system. Studies have found that when taken supplementally before bedtime, glycine can improve sleep in individuals who had been experiencing chronically poor sleep.[61]

Recommended dosage: 3 to 5 grams at night

Phosphatidylserine

This phospholipid, or a major component of all cell membranes, helps balance the body's cortisol levels. This is an excellent support if you find yourself perpetually stressed, and it often comes in a formula bundled with other stress response-mitigating herbs such as magnolia and ashwagandha.

Recommended dosage: 200 to 400 mg a day

Adaptogenic Herbs

Just like their name sounds, this class of plant helps your body adapt to the stresses of life. They're like thermostats — energizing you if you're tired and relaxing you if you're wired (in other words, they're "bidirectional"). Instead of just conking you out like a sedative, they smooth out your cortisol levels to where they should be when it's time to rest, helping bring your sympathetic and parasympathetic nervous systems back into balance. When taken regularly, they can help you fall asleep, stay asleep, and get better sleep. Two adaptogens in particular are great for sleep: ashwagandha and reishi, which you can buy in powdered form and stir into your evening tea.

Recommended dosages:

Ashwagandha: 500 to 1,000 mg per day of an extract standardized to 2.5–5 percent with anolides may reduce anxiety and help with sleep in people who are stressed or anxious

Reishi: 1 to 2 grams per day can help support sleep and the immune system

L-tryptophan

Your body converts this essential amino acid into serotonin, which helps regulate your mood (resolving anxiety, in particular) and sleep (especially improving how quickly you can fall asleep). You'll often see L-tryptophan in herbal sleep formulas. However, know that in some people, L-tryptophan can have a paradoxical effect, keeping them up instead.

Recommended dosage: 1 to 2 grams at night

Skullcap

A member of the mint family, this botanical has been used in traditional healing practices to address sleep issues and anxiety. We now know that skullcap stimulates gamma-aminobutyric acid (GABA), a neurotransmitter that has a calming effect on the nervous system.

Recommended dosage: 1 to 2 grams at night

Chinese and Ayurvedic Herbs

Traditional Chinese medicine and Ayurveda are traditional healing practices that have used medicinal herbs as part of their protocol for centuries. These herbal formulas are thoughtfully blended and prescribed with rhythm in mind—the herbs working in rhythm with one another, and the formula working in rhythm with your physiology. They're meant to be used over time in order to create a layered, cumulative effect that puts you back in sync, thereby addressing a wide range of health complaints. There are formulas that can be particularly beneficial for sleep, and we recommend working with a qualified practitioner to create a protocol that addresses your specific needs.

GABA

Gamma-aminobutyric acid (GABA) is a naturally occurring amino acid that works as a sort of bouncer in the brain, blocking or inhibiting brain signals in order to calm down the nervous system. This helps quell stress and feelings of anxiety or fear, while also encouraging relaxation and facilitating restful sleep. Sleep medications and anti-anxiety meds (like Valium, Lunesta, and Xanax) work by targeting the body's own GABA system to increase sedation and sleep, since low GABA activity is linked to insomnia and disrupted sleep. You can get GABA through your diet, particularly in fermented foods like kimchi, miso, and tempeh, as well as in black and oolong tea, but you can also supplement.

Recommended dosage: 300 to 660 mg at night

Valerian Root

This plant has been used to promote relaxation and sleep since ancient times and contains a number of compounds that may reduce anxiety and promote sleep, including valerenic acid, which has been found to inhibit the breakdown of GABA in the brain, resulting in feelings of calm and tranquility (the same way anti-anxiety medications and sleep meds work, but much safer). Research suggests that taking valerian root may improve the ability to fall asleep, as well as sleep quality and quantity.

Recommended dosage: 300 to 600 mg at night

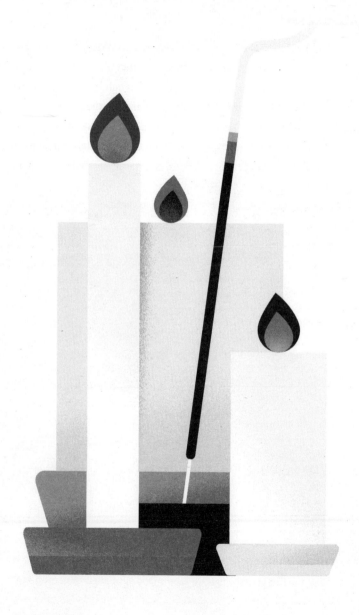

CHAPTER 7

SANCTUARY TO SLEEP

You've taken steps to heal underlying health issues that are affecting your sleep, adopt a rhythm-setting sleep schedule, and embrace new daily habits to achieve a better night's rest. While these actions will ultimately be the foundation of your success, we can't let you graduate from snooze school without a course in preparing your sleep environment.

Your nighttime surroundings play a significant role in your rhythm, in that they can either interfere with things like melatonin production and the restorative benefits of slow-wave sleep, or encourage them. Paying attention to factors like the temperature of your room, soothing smells, the quality of your bedding, or how in sync you are with your partner isn't just the stuff of fluffy magazine articles. Making your bedroom a sleep sanctuary also doesn't have to be complicated or expensive. With some very simple adjustments, you can create a space that's as relaxing as it is healing.

The ideal environment for sleep isn't unlike our first cave bedrooms — dark, cool, and quiet. Of course, we can do a little better than that by also making it extremely comfortable with a mattress that supports your joints and prevents aches and pains from keeping you awake, breathable bedding that doesn't trap too much heat, and pillows that not only do all of the above but also keep you breathing optimally and potentially address any snoring issues you may have. Add in some essential oils, candlelight, and white noise, and you've got yourself the perfect cocoon for welcoming and preserving sleep.

Disclaimer

The result of following the suggestions in this chapter will be a sleep refuge so scrumptiously relaxing that you'll want to spend as much time in there as possible. Don't be tempted! One of the keys to resting better at night is leaving your bed to two things: sleep and sex. But feel free to apply many of these tips to other rooms in your house—it can only benefit your health and happiness.

SET THE MOOD

As you read about in "Sync with the Sun" (page 74) and "Dim with the Dark" (page 78), the body relies on light cues to set its day-night rhythm. Quick recap: When you expose your light-sensor cells to artificial light at night, it delays the onset of melatonin, interferes with the quality and duration of your sleep, and throws off your sleep cycle. Which is why removing those sources of light from your bedroom is one of the most impactful ways you can improve your sleep. You'll find that these adjustments not only boost your sleep but also help create a relaxing environment that makes going to bed less of a chore and more of an indulgence.

Unplug Unnecessary Electronics in Your Bedroom.

Even those small blinking lights on your router, cable box, and surge protector are enough to inhibit melatonin production. If you can, move as many of those items out of your room, and replace any other light-producing electronics (especially that glaringly bright digital alarm clock) with either a low-fi unlit version or a tech-forward lamp that wakes you gently with light in the morning ("Light Time at the Right Time," page 77). By removing as many of these items as possible, you'll also be reducing the EMFs (electromagnetic fields) in your sanctuary, but more on that on page 192. And if it's not possible to move or cover light-generating electronics (black tape can come in handy for this), consider sleeping with an eye mask instead.

Hang Blackout Curtains

Unless you're living in a rural area with very little light pollution, chances are there's some kind of light coming in through your window. Light-blocking window treatments—even a simple roller shade that you can buy at the hardware store and easily hang yourself—is an effective way to make sure that you can reach ultimate bedroom cave status. If it's not possible to cover your windows, an eye mask is a suitable alternative.

Remember that when you block all light from the outside, you're also keeping out the important brain-stimulating dose of sunshine that comes in in the morning. Make sure you're diligent about throwing open the shades first thing, so your body's clock stays on track. Or if you sleep with an eye mask, consider investing in one that gradually exposes you to light, such as Illumy.

Read Like It's 1999

Reading in bed is one of life's great pleasures. If you're a bedtime reader, turn off your electronics (no excuses) and go old-school with a paper book, *not* an electronic one. Use a very small table lamp and the lowest watt amber bulb you can find. Keep in mind, though, that while getting swept up in a good novel may be just the thing after a long day, it's also important to be ready to cut yourself off for a proper bedtime.

If ditching your e-reader is a deal breaker, consider buying a blue-light filter or a pair of amber-tinted blue-blocker glasses, and keep the back light on your device as dim as possible without causing eye strain. Reading in a gently lit room as opposed to the pitch dark will also help with easing the burden on your eyes.

Get Melatonin-Mellowed

Keeping things dark in the bedroom is not just about after you turn off the light. You have to ease your body into sleep, which includes the two to three hours leading up to bedtime. For Neil, that used to mean lying in bed watching TV. After all, he grew up—like a lot of us— falling asleep watching TV on the sofa. When he moved his TV out of his bedroom, though, he was able to institute a screen-time curfew and spend time before bedtime relaxing in his bedroom without disruptive blue light.

Remember that lights brighter than a table lamp can mess with melatonin, so consider replacing harsh overhead lights with dimmer sources like candles (the flameless variety is great for anyone with kids or pets who are prone to knocking things over) or lamps. We're big fans of warm-light lamps that progressively dim as it gets closer to lights-out (like Casper's Glow Light and the Hatch Restore Tight), as well as Himalayan salt lamps, which give off a warm and gentle pink glow and are believed to help purify the air and balance electromagnetic radiation (both of which also improve sleep).

Gently Light Your Way

Flipping on the bathroom light in the middle of the night is a great way to send your sleep cycle reeling. Instead, try a nightlight with a low-watt red bulb, as red light is the easiest on your melatonin. Or add a flameless candle to a corner of the bathroom. And it pretty much goes without saying, but whatever you do, don't use your phone to find your way.

Make a Hydration Station

A sleep sanctuary hack that Neil discovered was keeping a glass of water on his bedside table. He, like many others, occasionally wakes up feeling thirsty but doesn't have the energy or will to get out of bed (not to mention the fact that getting up can be more disruptive if you have trouble falling back asleep). Having a glass at arm's reach means no lost sleep over feeling parched.

KEEP IT COOL

Your body cools at night and warms during the day, a natural ebb and flow that mirrors our circadian relationship with the sun. It's also functional—your body undergoes changes at night to ease you into sleep, including a drop in blood sugar and heart rate, both of which decrease your body and brain temperature. And because of science, we know that this makes a big difference in the quality of our sleep: A 2012 study confirmed that when we're too warm at night, it can lead to both delayed and disrupted sleep,[62] and people who sleep in hot environments can have elevated levels of cortisol in the morning, namely because a too-warm bedroom fights against the body's natural cooling-down process and throws off your sleep cycle. Insomnia has even been linked to a glitch in the body's heat-regulation cycles, meaning the body can't cool down when it wants to (a familiar side effect of pregnancy and menopause). People who sleep in cold environments, on the other hand, have been observed in studies to be more alert the next morning.

What experts say:

The optimal temperature range for your bedroom is 65°F to 68°F—although there are outliers who go as far as to say that 60°F, at least in the winter, is where it's at.

What we say:

Go for as cold as you can without feeling uncomfortable, and also keep the seasons in mind.

In the winter, give your thermostat a break (the efficient and environmentally friendly upside of your sleep-better protocol) by letting the temps in your house dip down. You can add more blankets to your bed, or wear socks, which is a more precise way to regulate your temperature. (You could also wear a hat, but we'd like to think we're more reasonable than that.)

In summer, however, don't crank up the AC. Instead, cool your room with a fan and by switching to more breathable sheets ("Make Your Bed," page 182). You'll also find that by adjusting your diet for your sleep protocol (especially cutting down on sugar and alcohol)—and by extension eliminating chronic inflammation and/or hormonal imbalances—you'll be helping to bring down your core temperature.

Add some tech:

Neil has been tracking the developments from companies like BedJet, Chillipad, and Ooler that make bed heating and cooling pads. They are also dual-sided, so if you share your bed with a partner, you can each have your own optimal microclimate.

For Better Sleep, Save the Planet

Among medical professionals, it's now widely accepted that there's a link between global warming and the rising frequency of health issues. As we use more and more fossil fuel-derived energy and the planet gets hotter, it affects our bodies' need to cool and contributes to chronic inflammation, which further raises the body's core temperature. It's a stark reminder that our internal environment is a direct reflection of our external environment—we can only be as healthy as our planet.

MAKE YOUR BED

If sleeping is one of the most—if not *the* most—important thing you can do for your health, then your bed, and all the stuff on it that you use to sleep, is pretty much the most important equipment you have. And not to toot our own horn, but one of us just so happens to be an expert on the topic. As the team at Casper likes to say: Think of your bed like an athlete would think of his or her gear—you wouldn't train for a marathon in the pair of sneakers you've had for the past 10 years, you wouldn't go to spin class wearing a pair of wool pants, and you wouldn't play football with protective pads that had gone shapeless and soft with wear. So why are you going to bed with a mattress that doesn't support your back, sheets that trap too much heat, and a pillow that leaves your neck unsupported and your airways partially blocked? There's really no excuse. Thanks to a number of great mattress and pillow manufacturers making their products available direct-to-consumer, as well as big-box retailers offering a wider selection of quality bedding, chances are that you can invest in your sleep wellness with minimal effort while staying within your budget.

When it comes to making your ultimate sleep-better bed, here's the gospel according to Neil:

The Mattress:

First, let's dispel one of the biggest myths when it comes to mattresses: *Firmness* and *support* are not the same thing. If your mattress was supposed to be as firm as the floor in order to best support your back, then you'd be better off sleeping on the floor. Lucky for you, that's not the case.

When searching for a supportive mattress, it's ideal to try it out for longer than just five minutes in the store. Your back muscles actually readjust to your new mattress over the first 35 to 45 days, co-evolving with your bed. And trying it out for that amount of time will also clue you in to whether your mattress has a comfortable microclimate (i.e., doesn't sleep too hot) and dampens movement from your partner, if applicable. (But you may not want a mattress that dampens too much movement—things like memory foam can be great for your back, but may not offer enough bounce for the other activities you enjoy in your bed.) So bottom line: You won't actually know whether a mattress is a good fit until you've spent about a month test-driving it.

And speaking of test-driving, you should absolutely think of buying a mattress the way you'd think of buying a car. You spend at least eight hours a day in your bed, far longer than you'd typically spend in your car, so consider that when prioritizing this investment. You don't necessarily need a handmade horsehair mattress to get the best night's sleep—the same way you don't need a Bugatti to get to the grocery store—but the Toyotas and Audis of mattresses are going to yield better results than something in the economy class. A cheaper mattress will probably not give you the support you need and will likely be made with closed-cell foam which, in addition to trapping hot air and creating a warmer microclimate, is not particularly healthy to be breathing in all night.

Which raises another great point: When it comes to buying a "healthier" mattress—or one that emits fewer VOCs (volatile organic compounds, or chemicals that have adverse health effects), be aware that a good amount of "greenwashing" exists in the mattress market. These are claims that are unregulated and often unfounded, such as calling a product "green" because it contains tea tree oil (we're still not sure how that makes for a better night's sleep) or putting a pretty picture of a green plant on a company website. A vast majority of mattresses are not certified organic because they contain some sort of polyurethane-based foam inside. If this is a concern to you, you can either find a mattress with official organic certification (such as Oeko-Tex Standard or

Certipure) or allow your mattress to air out for a day with the windows open before sleeping on it. In the case of mattresses that are compressed in the factory before being shipped to you, a majority of VOCs are pressed out before reaching you, but it can still be beneficial to air them out as they reinflate, especially if you consider yourself to be sensitive to any smells that may linger from production and shipping.

After 7 to 10 years—or whenever you notice that your mattress is no longer supportive or is sleeping hotter than usual (usually a result of all the organic materials we shed that our mattresses soak up)—do it all over again! In the meantime, consider using a breathable mattress protector—and even vacuuming your mattress occasionally—to keep it clean and relatively organic material–free.

The Pillows:

In addition to your mattress, a pillow is crucial for spinal alignment, which in turn leads to less aches and pains, which in turn leads to less interrupted sleep (not to mention better quality of life). When you lie on a pillow, it should support your neck and keep it in a straight line with your spine. Don't get hung up on finding a pillow for the "type" of sleeper you are (side, back, stomach)—what we've found in our research at Casper is that people on average switch sleeping positions about twenty times a night. Your pillow should support you no matter how you're sleeping on it.

There are a lot of options out there in terms of filling materials, and you have to weigh the pros and cons: Natural fibers (wool, kapok, buckwheat) can be more expensive and tend to not be as supportive as synthetics. Synthetics (memory foam, microfiber) are cheaper and can have really good support, but then again, it's synthetic—you're essentially sleeping with plastic next to your head (though, granted, you can find these pillows encased in natural and even organic materials). And then there's down, which makes for a quality product, but isn't hypoallergenic, which may be important to anyone with sensitivities to feathers.

Another thing to consider with a pillow is whether it's machine-washable. Your head is basically sweating into your pillow all night, every night (gross, but true), which then gets trapped in your pillow. Tossing it into the washing machine every so often is not a bad idea, especially if you're sensitive to things like dust and dander from pets. You could also use a pillow protector, but bear in mind that—like mattress protectors—anything meant to keep things out is also going to prevent optimal airflow.

> A great resource for finding unbiased reviews of the best bed-related gear is *Consumer Reports*.

The Sheets

First, let's dispel the myth of the 1,000-thread-count hotel collection sheets being the gold standard. That tight of a weave does nothing but trap hot air and humidity. You want to look for a lower thread count, ideally 200 to 400, which has a more open weave, allowing more air to circulate through the sheets. And always look for natural materials like linen, cotton, and silk. They sleep much cooler than synthetic materials, which trap heat and moisture and keep your core temperature from going down the way it's supposed to.

The Blankets

Think of your blankets like you do your clothes—layer! It's going to give you the most flexibility in reaching your maximum comfort throughout the night. Instead of going all-in on the biggest, fluffiest duvet with a heavy fill (which will also make you pretty warm), consider a lightweight duvet coupled with a quilt or cotton blanket (or two). Then you can add or subtract a layer as needed. In Europe, couples tend to have their own set of bedding so they can each create their own sleep climate. If you or your partner tends to sleep colder than the other, consider getting one large lightweight duvet and then a couple of smaller (i.e., twin-sized) blankets for one side. Whatever you choose, remember the same rule as above: Choose breathable natural fibers (cotton, linen, wool if you're not allergic) over synthetic.

And don't forget to change with the seasons. There's no rule that says you have to make your bed the same way year-round. You want lightweight breathability in the summer (like a thin cotton blanket or linen top sheet) and more thermal comfort in the winter, which is when the layered approach comes in handy.

Extra Credit: A Weighted Blanket

Weighted blankets have become very popular because of their potential to ease anxiety and insomnia, making it easier to fall asleep. They're designed to provide deep touch pressure—essentially creating the effect of a firm, comforting hug. This type of pressure has been shown to increase serotonin, which has a calming effect and is also the precursor to melatonin. Also, that feeling of being held can spark the production of oxytocin, the ultimate in feel-good hormones that can relieve pain and stress while supporting your immune system. All of this adds up to a better night's sleep and can be particularly helpful if you or your children are living with ADHD, autism, or sensory processing disorders.

Pull the Plug on Electric Blankets

They pose a fire risk, are made with health-damaging flame retardants, interfere with your body's nighttime temperature rhythm, and create continuous exposure to electromagnetic fields (or EMFs, which we'll talk about on p. 192)—all of which is bad news for your new nighttime goals.

CONSIDER SWINGING

We're talking about the G-rated version, that is. Two new studies suggest that our brains are evolutionarily programmed to respond to rocking. According to the findings, resting while rocking in a hammock helps people (both those who have historically had trouble with sleep and those who have not) fall asleep more quickly, reach deep sleep more expediently, sleep more soundly, and maintain deep sleep for a longer period of time. As an added cherry on top, they also wake up with improved long-term memory formation.

While the news that gently rocking is a powerful sedative isn't exactly *news* (just ask the parents of young babies and anyone who has trouble staying awake in the car), the researchers were able to explain why this happens: When you rhythmically swing while sleeping, it synchronizes the waves in the part of the brain that is involved in both sleep and memory consolidation. That kind of potent system-override may be just the thing if you're struggling with falling asleep, particularly as a jump start to your sleep-better journey, and for a dose of optimism that you can and will, in fact, sleep better again. If you have the room, consider adding a hammock in your backyard for a nap (page 100), or even to hit the refresh button with a night spent out in nature (pages 97–98). There are a number of options out there that come on a frame and don't require trees. Some retailers also sell hammocks and hammock "swings" that can be suspended from your ceiling with the help of a strong anchor.

SLEEP SOUND

We were designed to sleep in silence; after all, the world used to be a much quieter place. But now most of us are subject to noise pollution, whether it's coming from outside (garbage trucks, construction, traffic) or inside (your partner, neighbors, the dog). In order to create the ultimate sleep haven, you want to think about two things: removing disruptive sound and layering in soothing, sleep-promoting sound.

Creating Quiet

One of the simplest and least expensive ways to block out disruptive noise is to wear ear plugs. You can easily find some of the nice, squishy soft ones that most people find comfortable to sleep with. However, if that's not desirable or possible (as is the case of those of you who need to be able to hear at night, like new parents), try adding white noise. This gentle whooshing effect is made up of all the different frequencies of sound, making it ideal for masking other sounds. You can purchase a white noise machine (we like Dohm's version, which uses a fan to create a soft whooshing sound), download an app (this is especially great for travel), or you could just use a fan.

A Sleepy Soundtrack

Some people find it useful to replace environmental noise with more ambient sound, such as ocean waves, gongs, sound bowls, or falling rain. There's no right or wrong way to mix your own sleep beats, so long as you can successfully fall asleep and stay there.

Making Waves

A third option is to experiment with sound that synchronizes your brain waves with those of deepest relaxation and sleep. Called "binaural beats," these sounds are made by combining two slightly different frequencies, which prompts the brain to "tune" to a perceived single tone. This causes brain wave activity to slow, helping you to relax, feel less anxious, and by extension, fall asleep more easily and sleep more soundly. While there is new technology that layers these wavelengths under soothing sounds (such as those you can download from the Monroe Institute or apps such as Pzizz or Brain fm), you can also go to the original source of traditional sound healing. For centuries, people have used vibrational instruments—such as Aboriginal didgeridoos and Tibetan or Himalayan singing bowls—to induce a meditative state and "bathe" the body in reverberations that deliver a number of restorative benefits. You can download tracks of these sounds to listen to as you fall asleep (or meditate, page 113), or seek out a practitioner or studio who offers sound baths.

THE NEUROACOUSTIC BIOHACK

Increasingly we've been hearing about people using new technologies for stress reduction and smoother sleep onset, especially as looking to gadgets to supplement health and lifestyle protocols gets more popular. The first is called NuCalm, which claims to relax the brain and body within minutes. It's a hardware/software mashup that combines electromagnetic frequencies with patented binaural soundtracks referred to as "neuroacoustic software" to release your body from the grips of the stress response and enhance the amount of GABA available for your brain, both of which the body needs in order to successfully transition to sleep. By wearing a light-blocking mask, placing a small frequency-emitting disc on your inner wrist, and listening to NuCalm's proprietary songs or sounds, you are, as the company asserts, shifting the frequencies in your body while your brain entrains to deeply relaxed alpha and theta waves — similar, in theory, to how traditional Chinese medicine aims to reset frequencies or qi in the body in order to promote healing shifts. After some experimentation with the technology ourselves, we both felt somewhat more relaxed. We ultimately agreed that it was a worthwhile consideration if you're interested in a tech-assisted boost to your stress management and sleep.

On the less expensive side of the spectrum is the Fisher Wallace Stimulator, which has been cleared by the FDA for the treatment of depression, anxiety, and insomnia. Using electrodes that you affix to the sides of your head for 20 minutes while you relax, it claims to stimulate serotonin production and alpha wave production while lowering cortisol.

Melodic Mornings

Consider incorporating gentle music or sounds into your wake-up routine too. A recent study found that when participants woke up to pleasant music, they were more alert, less groggy, and even less clumsy than those who were jolted awake by the sound of more harsh alarm tones.[63]

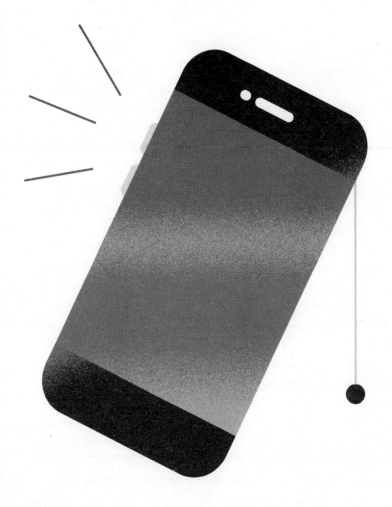

GIVE AN EFF ABOUT EMFs

A powerful way to help your sleep and health is to unplug. It is scientific fact that radiation from anything that uses or moves electricity and radio frequencies—including our Wi-Fi routers, Bluetooth devices, smartphones, smart refrigerators, smart cars, and even smart meters (yes, including your sleep tracker, but we'll come back to that)—is biologically disruptive. That's because these devices emit EMFs, or electromagnetic fields. EMFs act on the body similarly to the radiation of light, stimulating your cells to communicate and behave in certain ways. But like artificial light, these invisible manmade frequencies have the ability to "stress out" and ultimately damage your cellular function. No thanks to the omnipresence of our wireless technology, EMFs do this day and night.

Medicine is just beginning to understand just how dysregulating EMF exposure can be. However, studies already show that there is a clear connection between wireless radiation and detriments to our health, including headaches, difficulty focusing, anxiety, depression, fatigue, aches and pains, and irritability, as well as even more concerning effects such as structural and functional changes to the reproductive system, learning and memory deficits, neurological disorders, genetic damage, and cancer. The World Health Organization's International Agency for Research on Cancer (IARC) classified radio-frequency radiation as a Group 2B "Possible Carcinogen," though ongoing research will most likely upgrade this designation. Most recently, hundreds of scientists from more than 40 countries in Europe have signed a petition to call for the European Union to halt the rollout of the 5G network because of serious concerns over the effect it will have on people, plants, and animals.[64]

It should come as no surprise then that when it comes to sleep, EMFs are ultimately bad news. Because EMFs are an emerging concern, there has not yet been ample research conducted in this specific area of our health, but studies have found that exposure can decrease melatonin production. We also know that the body is most vulnerable to these stressful frequencies at night, as they interrupt the essential rest and repair functions happening at that time. And if your receptor cells are being fed information besides what's coming from the big, bright boss in the sky, it will most likely scramble your sleep frequencies too. But even though we don't yet have ample data to say definitively how these frequencies are affecting the body when it's trying to sleep, we can say that any steps you can take to decrease your exposure will help.

How to Unplug from EMFs

We can't eliminate all of our EMF exposure because some of it comes from relatively uncontrollable sources like communication towers and the electric wiring in your walls. But you can at least decrease the amount of radiation interacting with your body at night by following this advice:

- Turn off your phone, or at the very least put it on airplane mode.
- Don't charge your phone on your nightstand overnight. If you have to do it in your bedroom, keep it at least 6 feet from your bed.
- Turn off your Wi-Fi router.
- If your laptop must be in the same room as you, turn it off or at least disable your wireless connectivity.
- Keep any electronic devices in your room at least six feet away from your bed.

- Sleep on a mattress without metal springs. They can potentially magnify EMFs.
- If your bed shares a wall with a circuit breaker or major appliance, consider finding another spot for it.

What about My Sleep Tracker or App?

EMFs unfortunately don't make exceptions for technology that helps us sleep. It comes down to purpose over perfection. Our take is that you should go with whatever helps you sleep best now, with the goal of ultimately unplugging. Use sleep trackers and apps to help you get off to a strong start, then consider taking a break or removing them from your protocol. A great way to offset this additional EMF exposure is to add an earthing regimen (Feel the Earth Move, page 97).

CLEAR THE AIR

There is a link between the quality of air you breathe and the quality of your sleep—exposing yourself to pollution, particularly at night, can lead to lower sleep efficiency. Air pollution irritates your airways, causes congestion, and triggers allergies, which inhibits how well the body can breathe deeply and rhythmically, relax, and receive oxygen (one reason why there's a connection between air pollution and sleep apnea). Researchers also think it's possible that air particulates can get into the bloodstream and affect the regulation of sleep in the brain. While this thinking is still in the "association" stage versus "cause and effect," we do know that air quality plays a significant role in our health, which has downstream ramifications on our sleep.

Studies have shown that indoor air can, shockingly, be *two to five times* more polluted than outdoor air. Household cleaning products, cosmetics, and off-gassing from things like our carpeting, bedding, and furniture (aka volatile organic compounds or VOCs) all contribute airborne chemicals that muck up our immediate environment. To make sure that your sleep retreat is as beneficial as possible, take steps to give your air a detox:

- Whenever possible, open the windows for fresh outside air.
- Add air-filtering plants. Indoor plants can absorb pollutants (including VOCs) through their leaves and roots.
- Invest in a high-quality air purifier. Look for one that removes more than 99 percent of airborne contaminants that are larger than 0.3 microns.
- Run a humidifier. This won't remove toxins, but it can improve air quality and will add more moisture to the air, which helps to boost beneficial ionic elements (read more about this below). A humidifier can also help you breathe better at night, decrease the chances of catching a cold or other bugs, and wake up feeling less dried out in the morning.
- Don't introduce toxins in the first place. Opt for bedding and other bedroom textiles like curtains and rugs that are made from natural fibers, furniture that's made from natural materials (wood or metal versus plastic or MDF, a wood composite), and nontoxic cleaning agents without synthetic fragrances.

Clean Burn

Candles are a great way to introduce warm, calming light without throwing off your rhythm. But not all candles are created equal. Many conventional products release a number of chemicals when burned, which can further aggravate respiratory issues, among other health concerns. Paraffin- and petroleum-derived waxes are heavy on the toxins when burned, even when considered "premium" grade. And synthetic fragrances are known allergens and can contain phthalates (chemicals that can alter the functioning of your hormones, a process known as endocrine disruption). Look for a candle that's 100 percent soy or beeswax and made with naturally derived essential oils. Or skip the scent altogether—beeswax candles have a pleasing, subtle honey-like smell.

ION MAN

Flushing your cells with oxygen isn't the only benefit of breathing in fresh air. When we take air in, we also welcome charged ions, which invigorate our cells. This essentially creates an electric current that allows our nervous system to send signals through the body, affecting how we move, think, feel, and sleep. A disruption in that current can lead to a breakdown in that communication chain and ultimately illness. Active ions also help clean the air by oxidizing mold, fungi, parasites, and toxic chemical gases. They also bind to dust, pollen, and pet dander, making them larger particles that are easier to filter.

Movement and moisture boost ionic charge—think about how revitalized you feel after just breathing near oceans, rivers, waterfalls, and mountains. But if air stops moving, it can get stagnant and the ions start to lose their charge. Easily enough, though, all you need to do is get the air moving again by opening the window or turning on a fan. You could also invest in an air ionizer, especially for winter months when it's more difficult to get fresh air flowing.

GET SCENTERED

What you add to the air of your sleep sanctuary can be just as impactful as what you take away. Smell is a powerful sense that communicates directly with your memory and emotion centers of your brain. The ancient practice of using scent to heal, now called aromatherapy, is the original mind-body therapy and has been studied extensively for its stress-relieving, pain-reducing, mood regulating benefits A body of research has shown that essential oils—concentrated oil derived from various parts of a plant—can also improve sleep quality and provide relief from disrupted sleep. This smell-good sleep aid can't rewire your sleep rhythm on its own without other lifestyle shifts, but it's a very useful tool for encouraging your body to adapt to your new cycle.

Soporific Scents

No matter how much research backs the power of these oils (and there's quite a bit), choosing the right one for you is not an exact science. You simply have to smell a few and see which you like best. The winner is the correct prescription.

lavender
geranium
jasmine
rose
vanilla
ylang ylang
sandalwood[†]
citrus[†]

†These scents can be calming to some people but stimulating to others.

How to Use Essential Oils

Diffuse

Essential oil diffusers vaporize the oils and fill your room with a subtle but effective scent, since the vaporizing process makes the oils easier for you to inhale and absorb. This is not the same as adding a few drops of oil to a humidifier; doing so will start to degrade the plastic bits of your humidifier. Instead, you could put a drop or two on a cotton ball and put it into the vapor outlet. Other expert tips include not diffusing for more than 30 minutes (since it could become overstimulating), and being sensitive to your pets' reactions (not all tolerate oils well, especially cats, who don't have the liver enzyme needed to break down certain types of compounds).

Mist

Combine 4 to 5 drops of essential oil with a ½ cup of water, add to a spray bottle or atomizer, and spritz around your room and over your linens. Err on the side of caution when spraying the tops of your pillows; most skin doesn't like spending that much time with the oils.

Dab

You can apply essential oils to pressure points such as the wrists or behind the ears, or chakras such as the heart and the third eye. Just make sure to dilute these very concentrated and potentially irritating oils in carrier oils, such as coconut, jojoba, almond, or olive.

Bathe

Combine your nightly aromatherapy with your pre-snooze soak ("Take a Warm Bath," page 87). Add a few drops of your oil to warm bathwater, inhale, exhale, *aaaah*.

REDEFINE PILLOW TALK

If you share your bed with someone at night, then they too are a part of your sleep sanctuary. Actually, you'd ideally be part of *each other's* sleep sanctuary, partaking in the same habits and behaviors that add up to a good night's rest for both of you. But that can be easier said than done: As Neil learned from talking to thousands of couples looking to buy a mattress, a bed is often the closest proximity couples share with each other. And everyone has their own nighttime quirks (tossing and turning, snoring), preferences (all the blankets, none of the blankets), and habits (television to fall asleep, laptop in bed, up early for the gym).

It's no wonder that a recent survey found that nearly a third of American couples are interested in a "sleep divorce," or prefer to sleep separately from their partners. Ten percent said they've had an earlier relationship that actually ended over sleep issues. We, obviously, are Team Sleep all the way and support whatever it takes to get the night-time goods, but we'd rather see couples address the fundamental sleep issues that are driving them apart. Simply reading the first two chapters of this book together may be enough to get your partnership in sync. Just in case, though, we've included below some common issues that come up for bedfellows.

While we can offer up potential solutions, you need to be the ones having an open and honest conversation about what your respective needs are for sleep, then create an environment to make that happen. Try being open to new ideas, even if they seem strange at first—if it's the difference between sleeping poorly for the rest of your life or trying something new, it's worth talking about. You might just find a little more rest—and a little more heat—between the sheets.

Problem 1:

Not having the same sleep rhythm. One of you thrives on late-night productivity (or just catching up on TV), while the other likes to turn in early. One likes to start the day early while the other can't function before 10 a.m. Different chronotypes—or genetically coded preferences for when to sleep and wake—are a real thing ("Embrace Your Chronotype," page 71), but as you read in Chapter 4, there are ways to adjust your sleep rhythms so that they're at least a little more in tune with one another. The more you both can commit to consistent sleep and wake times that coincide with the day-night cycle, the more in sync you'll be.

Problem 2:

Not having the same sleep hygiene. Luckily, this book is the perfect resource (if we do say so ourselves) for arguing the case for getting more vitamin Z. Share with your partner some of the points from Chapter 1 (particularly from "The Out-of-Rhythm Body," page 26) that may resonate with them. Or better yet, encourage them to read the book themselves. You both can then compare the sleep-better habits that sound best/most relevant and create a common sleep-better protocol.

Problem 3:

Snoring. Gone are the days of suffering in silence (or in this case, chainsaw sound effects), or straight-up kicking your partner out of bed (or getting kicked out). There are tons of great gadgets on the market that help with snoring; head to "Shush Your Snoring" (page 88) and take your pick. And as also mentioned in that section, there's a very good chance that the dietary changes you or your partner make from Chapter 6 (especially ditching sugar and dairy and cutting back on alcohol) will significantly decrease the disruption.

Problem 4:

Running hot or cold. It's completely unrealistic to expect that you and your partner will benefit from the same microclimate. While we all do better sleeping in cooler temps, some of us love the feeling of cozy sweats and a fluffy duvet while others would rather sleep in the nude with nothing but a light top sheet. If you're not a couple that shares the love for the same type of bedding, consider doing what the Europeans do: split it up. Many couples choose to push together two twin beds, which they can outfit separately with linens, making for two different microclimates. This can also be helpful if one of you struggles with snoring and wants to have a mattress that elevates their head without disturbing the other party. Alternatively, you could make the bed with one large, light blanket, then use twin-sized blankets to layer on just one side.

Problem 5:

Too-tight quarters. Spooning aside, we need space when we sleep. This is mainly because sleeping in close proximity to another body keeps the bed microclimate warmer, plus knocking knees in the middle of the night isn't exactly restful—which goes double if you or your partner is a restless sleeper. We get that not everyone can easily upgrade to a bigger bed, but consider this one more option that may give you some nighttime respite.

Problem 6:

Arguing. Your mother was right—you should never go to bed angry. Our sleep suffers from toxicity, which includes the emotional turbulence of fighting with your partner. Experiencing anger and frustration in the evening stimulates the sympathetic nervous system and stress response, which keeps too much high-alert cortisol in your system when it should be saturated with yawn-inducing melatonin. Do whatever you have to do to make peace, whether it's talking things out, journaling, or doing breathwork. Or just get angry in the morning instead...

DON'T BLAME IT ON THE DOG

Sleeping with your cat or dog (or other sizeable pet) in the bed is sweet and calming, but if your creature has a tendency to take over the bed and disrupt your sleep or otherwise keep you from getting comfortable, then it's time to reconsider your priorities. Especially if you're prone to being woken up at night (and *double* especially if you have trouble falling back asleep once you're up), it may be best to remove this variable. It's not like there have been studies on the topic—at least not to our knowledge—and there's not much more to say, but in short: If your sleep sucks, Fido or Fluffy should go. At least for a little while. Sorry, Fido and Fluffy. Consider buying them a nice bed of their own—some companies (like Casper) offer ones that take support and pressure relief into consideration as much as they do for mattresses for humans.

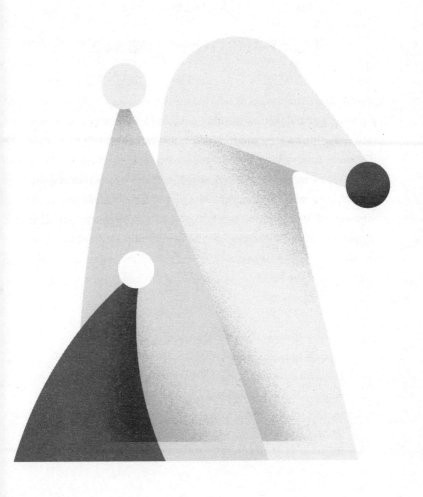

CHAPTER 8

SLEEP THROUGH THE AGES

From the time we're born, our sleep is constantly evolving. The number of hours we spend sleeping each night and how we cycle through the stages of sleep, which is known as our "sleep architecture," looks different as we transition from being babies to being young children, then adolescents, teenagers, adults, and finally seniors. But even though our sleep goals might be different in terms of how much time we're spending in bed, and our physiological needs change, we all have two things in common:

- We're all better off with more and better sleep. For kids, it directly impacts mental and physical development and can support better grades, healthier relationships, and more resilient emotional coping down the road. For older adults, it's essential for keeping the mind sharp and the body strong and illness-free.
- We can all take the same basic path to get back to that place. Rhythm is still the name of the game, no matter what age you or your kids are.

This chapter is dedicated to groups that deserve additional focus and guidance when it comes to their sleep: babies (and their parents), young children, adolescents, teenagers, and seniors. Our recommendation is to use the preceding sections as a baseline for understanding why sleep is critically important and the basics for what contributes to better nighttime rest. Then, you can layer in these specific recommendations as they pertain to you, your children, or your parents.

Seniors

One of the biggest misconceptions among more "seasoned" sleepers is that they don't need as much nighttime rest as they did when they were younger. Unfortunately, the pattern you start to see in people older than 65 of short, interrupted, or difficult-to-get-there sleep is not reflective of the fact that your sleep needs decline when you get older. In reality, the recommendation for how much sleep you should be getting is still seven to eight hours a night. So if you experience insomnia (as about 44 percent of the elderly population does[65]) or have difficulty falling asleep or staying asleep for the duration of the night (Harvard Medical School researchers have confirmed that is related to age), this is not an indication that your body is just doing what nature intended. On the contrary: It's your body asking you to pay more attention to your sleep.

And it is critical that you do pay attention because the worse you sleep, the more the aging process accelerates. That includes degeneration of the mind (dementia, Alzheimer's), as well as degeneration of the body. Getting a good night's sleep is one of your best defenses against aging quickly. The good news is that a number of the recommendations in this book speak directly to the kind of specialized support that your sleep needs.

Why Does Aging Affect Sleep?

> **Your sleep architecture,** or the amount of time you spend in each phase of sleep, shifts with age. Most notably, older adults spend more time in the lighter stages of sleep than in deep

sleep. This can make it more difficult to stay asleep, and also explains why the body is performing its nightly reparative processes less efficiently.

Your circadian rhythm also begins to change, causing many older people to get sleepier earlier in the evening and wake earlier in the morning. It's a pattern called "advanced sleep phase syndrome." We still don't know why this happens, but it's suspected that it has something to do with falling out of rhythm with natural light cues.

Your brain also plays a role, owing to the fact that its neurological receptors, which connect with sleep-signaling chemicals, get weaker. Basically, your brain has a harder time figuring out when you're tired.

Your medical conditions and the medications used to treat them have also been identified as the major cause behind sleep disturbances in older sleepers.[66] Health problems like arthritis, GERD, and restless leg syndrome can cause discomfort that makes it harder to fall asleep. An enlarged prostate will also cause you to wake frequently and go to the bathroom. And certain prescription drugs (especially those that treat heart problems, blood pressure, and asthma) in addition to over-the-counter meds (like cold and headache medications) can interfere with falling and staying asleep.

Your habits throughout the day are another major culprit. Napping for too long or too late in the day, relying on caffeine for a second wind in the afternoon or evening, eating too close to bedtime, and not moving your body throughout the day can all throw off the rhythms that need to be reinforced for a successful bedtime.

Your Sleep Solution:

Pay special attention to the following sections in the book when creating your sleep-better protocol. We also recommend taking the "What's Your Not-Sleeping Type?" quiz (page 45) in order to assess any other underlying roadblocks that might be making your sleep issues worse.

End Social Jet Lag Turbulence (page 68)

Sync with the Sun (page 74)

Have a Powering-Down Practice (page 85)

To Nap or Not to Nap? (page 100)

Move to Sleep (page 102)

Loosen Up (page 120)

Eat in Rhythm (page 137)

Curb Caffeine (page 148)

Edit Your Meds (page 153)

BABIES

There are entire books dedicated to helping babies sleep through the night as they learn how to transition from sleep cycle to sleep cycle. As many books as there are out there, there are just as many philosophies about which approach is best for doing just that (the cry-it-out method, the no-cry method, the change-it-up-every-night-in-desperation method). We'll stay in our lane here and keep our noses out of that conversation, but we will weigh in on another important issue if you are a new parent: *your* sleep.

First, let us offer a little peace of mind: It's a normal human condition occasionally to be sleepless, and at your age you're resilient enough that this hiccup isn't going to cause long-term issues. Also, 70 percent of babies sleep through the night by the time they're nine months old—this won't last forever.

Now let's get you sleeping as best you can. We might not be able to get your baby to sleep (sorry), but we can give you this advice, which will hopefully empower you to take the best possible care of yourself. Remember, a (relatively) well-rested parent is a happier, healthier, saner parent.

- **Forget everything we said about syncing with the sun.** You're now in survival mode and need to get rest whenever you can. Instead of thinking of sleep as happening only between night and morning, accept any sleep you can get on a 24-hour basis, no matter what time of day.
- **Sleep when baby sleeps.** Seriously. Put down the laundry, leave the dishes in the sink, and get your butt in bed. Even if it's only 20 minutes, that's enough to give you a temporary reboot.
- **Accept help.** Lean on your partner, friends, and family to look after the baby while you rest or at the very least tackle those aforementioned dishes. If you're able to, hire a postpartum doula, someone who is trained to give both you *and* your baby support. If you're breastfeeding, consider asking a lactation consultant about transitioning to a bottle for some feedings.
- **Keep the lights dim.** When you have to get up in the night for a feeding or diaper change, use soft, warm light instead of bright overhead or even lamp light, which can disrupt your melatonin production and make it difficult for both you and your baby to fall back asleep. Candles can be great for this, especially LED versions that won't pose a fire hazard in case you doze off.
- **Don't forget the sleep sanctuary basics.** This goes for both you and your baby—a dark, cool, quiet room not only facilitates sleep, it also triggers the body into realizing that it's

time to sleep when you make these attributes a habitual part of
your sleep environment.

■ **Loop in your ped.** If you suspect that your baby's sleep
schedule is being affected by an underlying health condition
(acid reflux, for example), talk to your pediatrician.

Young Children

In many ways, the sleep habits that start at this age translate into better
sleep hygiene once your child is an adolescent, teenager, and even
adult. None of the advice here is particularly specific to being a young
child—rather they're universal sleep-better guidelines. When learned
and embraced early, they pave the way for a lifetime of better sleep.

■ **Teach your kids that sleep is for superheroes.** It's not too
early to start explaining why sleep is so important (especially when
prompted with "I don't want to go to bed!"). You don't have to
start unpacking the science, but just as you teach kids that eating
healthy food makes their brains smart and bodies strong, you can
let them know that so too does a good night's sleep.

■ **Stop using sleep as a punishment.** Many of us have been
there—"Cut it out or I'll send you up to bed!" Instead of
messaging that sleep means not getting to do something more
enjoyable, let your kids know that sleep is something special and
rewarding that we *get* to do every night.

■ **Maintain a regular and consistent sleep schedule.** This
includes during longer breaks from school, when the tendency
is to completely disregard the habits created during the school
year. There is of course some flexibility, but keep in mind that
it's the consistency that will beget better sleep—and make
transitioning back to school less of a struggle.

■ **Create a relaxing bedtime routine.** Just as you need to
power down, so do your kids. They shouldn't go from running

around the house at full tilt to having light's out. Instead, slowly wind down with turning off electronics (yes, it's just as stimulating for them as it is for you), dimming the lights, a bath, and a story or two. Embrace this time as a run-up to your own bedtime routine and winding down for the night.

- **Kids need sleep sanctuaries too.** Just like you, they need a dark, cool, quiet, unstimulating environment to sleep in. Essential oils can also be helpful for creating bedtime calm, particularly lavender. For older kids, consider keeping their rooms electronics-free, including televisions and computers.
- **Dig into diet.** The same guidelines apply for kids as they do for us — things like sugar and caffeine are pretty much the worst things you can ingest when it comes to not only sleep but overall health too. Monitor how much sugar is lurking in those just-for-kids snacks and other treats, and remember that sodas, in addition to being laden with sugar, tend to contain caffeine as well.

ADOLESCENTS AND TEENS

Sleep for young people in this group has been described as the "perfect storm." That's because the need for a good night's rest is just as important for their development and wellbeing as it was when they were children, yet the number of factors that can encroach on their sleep multiplies exponentially. Throw in the fact that many parents, teachers, young people themselves, and even pediatricians assume that the resulting decline in healthy sleep is "just a part of growing up," and you can see why trouble starts to brew.

In reality, adolescents and teenagers need far more sleep than you'd think — 9 to 12 hours for kids aged 6 to 12, and 8 to 10 hours for teenagers 13 to 18. If your kid is consistently getting less (which researchers suggest they most likely are), then they're exposing themselves to the same physiological detriments that you are when subjecting your body to chronic sleep deficit: foggy thinking, difficulty with learning and memory, lethargy, moodiness, depression, anxiety, reduced ability to handle stress, lowered decision-making abilities, hormone fluctuations, weight gain, and increased risk of caffeine and/or nicotine use. That's definitely *not* what you want to be throwing in the mix on top of the standard-issue concerns your preteen or teen is facing.

And no, your kid staying up to study isn't ultimately what's going to get them ahead. Researchers at MIT found a strong relationship between students' grades and how much sleep they're getting, with bedtime consistency also making a difference.[67]

Some of the most common causes for sleep deficits in adolescents and teens include:

- **Irregular sleep patterns.** Most adolescents and teens are getting barely enough sleep during the week, then trying to make up for it on the weekends. But as you now know, that's only a recipe for sleep-rhythm and sleep-quality disaster.
- **Biological sleep pattern shift.** There is a natural tendency to go to bed later as kids reach adolescence, but that doesn't necessarily mean it's optimal. Unfortunately, because of early school start times, a later bedtime isn't conducive to getting a proper night's sleep. This new circadian rhythm—especially when combined with social jet lag, blue-light exposure, and late-day caffeine consumption—sometimes leads kids to believe that just because they have trouble falling asleep at a healthy hour (before 11 p.m.) doesn't mean they should have to.
- **Social stigma of early bedtimes.** What kind of self-respecting, rule-bucking, too-cool-for-school kid has a bedtime? (The ones whose parents instilled in them the

importance of sleep for their wellbeing, smarts, and general peace of mind.)

- **Increased technology use.** If they're not watching television, many kids are on their tablets, computers, or phones well into the dark hours. As you now know, that blue-light exposure is extremely detrimental to melatonin production, making it even more difficult for them to fall asleep at a reasonable hour.

Better Sleep 101

When it comes to helping your adolescent or teen get better sleep, we realize you're up against a lot of factors, many of which you may not be able to change (at least not in the short term, in the case of school start times). You'll notice that many of these suggestions are the same as what we recommend for adults—all the more reason to make sleeping better a family affair.

- **Set a consistent bedtime.** We know it sounds kind of... intense, especially for older kids. But studies show that adolescents whose parents enforced a bedtime of 10 p.m. or earlier were less likely to experience depression or suicidal ideations than those who could stay up until midnight.[68] Work with your kid to create a realistic schedule that works for them and their schoolwork, and do your best to keep it consistent, including on the weekends. Extra sleep-in time on Saturday and Sunday can make it more difficult to get in bed by a healthy time come Monday.
- **Consider a nap.** If schedules allow, having your kid take a quick 20- to 30-minute nap immediately following school could help chip away at their overall sleep deficit, as well as eliminate any perceived need to consume caffeine in order to study that night.

- **Limit tech in the evening.** A European study found that by reducing the exposure to light-emitting screens on phones, tablets, and computers, adolescents can improve their sleep quality and reduce symptoms of fatigue, lack of concentration, and irritability after just one week.[69] Consider implementing a "media curfew," turning off the Wi-Fi in the evening, or having everyone in the family leave their devices at the same charging station overnight. And definitely get the electronics out of their room—computer included.

- **Talk to your kid.** Break down the benefits of good sleep and the significant drawbacks of not getting enough. Point out that kids who sleep for just 60 extra minutes get higher grades, feel less distracted or overwhelmed in class, and maintain a better mood than those who don't. Or that more sleep makes it easier to maintain clear skin and an ideal weight—whatever might resonate with your kid. Share the tidbits that you learn about in this book and help your kid navigate common pitfalls, like subpar nutrition and stimulant use.

- **Be in it together.** Just like kids are more likely to eat their vegetables if they see you doing it too, they are much more likely to adopt healthier sleep habits if you're modeling them. Plus, by following your own sleep-better protocol, you'll innately be able to include the entire family, whether it's beginning to dim the lights early in the evening, closing the kitchen to late-night grazing, encouraging a family-wide tech turn-off, or playing some relaxing music.

The School Snafu

A recent report by the U.S. Centers for Disease Control and Prevention shed stark light on the fact that most kids aren't getting the sleep they need. More than half of the middle-school children assessed were getting less than the recommended amount, and when it came to high school, that number jumped to 75 percent.[70] While there are a number of factors that explain why kids in this demographic are chronically sleep deprived, there's one that's more insidious than all of them combined: school.

As kids go through puberty, their circadian rhythm shifts to look more like an adult's, making it more difficult to go to bed as early as they did as kids. But they still need, on average, 10 hours of sleep, and, unlike most of us, they have to be up and ready to perform by 7 or 8 a.m. This would be like us having to wake up at 3 a.m. and start working at 4 a.m. Very few kids are ready to learn before 8:30 a.m., and yet a poll by the National Sleep Foundation found that 87 percent of high school students have to do just that.

This circadian nightmare isn't without consequences. Kids who start their first class of the day before 8 a.m. perform worse in school for the rest of the day than those with a later start time. They experience more emotional and behavioral problems, have worse impulse control and decision-making skills, and they're more likely to drive while drowsy.

(Which is just as dangerous as drunk driving—there are 6,400 fatal drowsy-driving-caused crashes each year, and teens are typically involved in half of them.[71]) These sleep-deprived kids are also more likely to use tobacco and alcohol and less likely to excel academically or athletically.

But there's a solution: When schools around Minneapolis, Minnesota, moved their high schools' 7:15 and 7:25 a.m. start times to 8:30 or 8:40 a.m., teachers and school administrators noted that attendance improved and tardiness decreased, as did trips to the school nurse. Students were more alert in class, they were less likely to be disciplined, and the schools had an overall "calmer" atmosphere. Other districts have reported similar findings, as well as higher standardized test scores and fewer car crashes.

This is why many health and education experts as well as a number of organizations are pushing for later school start times in middle and high schools. If you're a parent, consider making noise—get other parents involved in the cause, talk to the school board. Show them the data of what happens to our kids when we mess with their sleep. Luckily, there's a growing precedent for this shift, and if we all keep pushing in our respective districts, we can make a difference that helps kids everywhere.

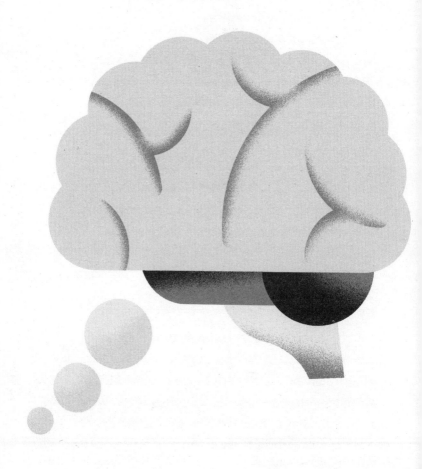

CHAPTER 9

IN YOUR DREAMS

Even though we think of sleep as "powering down," our brains are doing anything but that when we get shut-eye. Without any incoming stimulation or thoughts, the brain uses this valuable free time to perform maintenance and admin—cleansing, consolidating memories, and imprinting new information. And we now know that dreaming is an important part of these nocturnal activities.

Scientists used to think that dreams were just a by-product of the brain's nighttime regimen. However, new research has shown us that dreaming actually serves a number of important functions, especially for our learning and memory. But if you're not sleeping well (not reaching deep sleep or waking up multiple times a night), then you're missing out on one more essential tool that your brain needs in order to keep you healthy and sharp.

Even though you may not know whether you're dreaming on a regular basis (we dream at all stages of sleep, not just REM, and don't necessarily remember all the content), it's safe to say that if you're consistently cycling through all four stages of sleep without regular interference (meaning you're getting a full, restful night's sleep), then you're going to reap the benefits of dreams. The advantages of nighttime dreaming are numerous.

Dreams help us store memories and the things we've learned.

The brain reactivates and consolidates newly received memories and information tidbits while we sleep, and researchers have seen that this process is directly reflected in the content of our dreams.[72] But some experts believe that dreams aren't just *reflecting* what we need to know and remember, they're actively cataloging it. Their findings suggest that our dreams are a sort of virtual reality experience as we witness this memory processing.[73] Experiments in both animals and humans support the theory that our dreams are like a "rehearsal" of that new information, allowing our brain to put it into practice and actively organize and consolidate the material.[74]

Dreams help process our emotions.

Recent research suggests that we're more likely to dream about emotionally intense experiences, and the theta brain waves during REM sleep are one way in which the brain consolidates those memories. This has led some researchers to examine how REM sleep plays a role in trauma recovery and mood regulation, owing to its hand in processing difficult experiences.

Even nightmares have benefits.

Nightmares occur most frequently in REM sleep, but unlike lucid dreams, these intense, often unwelcome imaginings happen with decreased prefrontal cortex activity, meaning there's less emotional control and a more overwhelming sense of arousal. Researchers now believe that these experiences are the brain's way of preparing us for when bad things happen, like an emotional "dress rehearsal." It's almost as though the mind is anticipating bad things happening, and then trying out solutions. Some experts believe that this is a defense mechanism rooted in our earliest days—if something bad happened once, there was a chance it could happen again. So having a recurring nightmare of that event could keep you on guard.

At the very least, dreams offer another way of looking at things.

Dreams don't just simply replay what we've experienced or learned, they also create brand-new mashups and free associations between what we've seen and what we know. As a result, our dreams offer a portal into our deepest, most unfettered creativity, as well as to new approaches to problem-solving. This is most evident in the testimonies of famous artists and thinkers who credit their dreams with inspiring some of their greatest creations, like Paul McCartney and the melody for "Yesterday" or Dmitri Mendeleev and the structure for the periodic table of elements.

What Your Dreams Say about Your Sleep

The nature of your dreams can lend insight into what cycle of sleep you're dreaming in:

Stage 1: During this fuzzy, foggy time just before you drift off or wake up, dreams are usually short but feel vivid and visceral, like having the sensation of "falling" to sleep. Because you're still in a semi-awake state, these dreams often incorporate real-world content like noises you're actually hearing (your alarm, a siren outside).

Stage 2: In this lighter stage of sleep, dreams usually include pieces of real-life events from the day. They're often described as being "thought-like," as though you're merely processing different ideas while you sleep. As you revisit stage 2 sleep throughout the night, your dreams will gradually get longer and more vivid.

Stage 3: Even though your brain is still active during deep sleep, your dreams are typically the least vivid during this stage as your brain tends to memory processing and cognition renovation.

REM: This is the stage of sleep that's most frequently associated with dreams. Dreams that occur during these more "active" peaks in your sleep cycle are the ones you usually remember most: they're typically the longest, most vivid, and most bizarre. (We also get a lot of REM sleep in the morning, so the timing is more conducive to remembering these dreams.) Also, this is the stage of sleep when the emotional parts of the brain are most active, which is what experts suspect makes our REM dreams feel more poignant and affecting.

DREAM FACTORY

Different parts of the brain contribute to different types of dreams, giving them each unique qualities:

The cortex: This is where most of our memories are stored, and it's the main content creator for our dreams. It explains why our dreams are strangely autobiographical and pull from seemingly random snippets of things we've seen or done.

The sensory cortices: This audio/visual storehouse is also active in providing dream details, which is why some dreams seem like they come with their own unique sounds and, less frequently, smells.

The motor cortex: Responsible for controlling our movements when we're awake, this part of the brain also kicks in at night and contributes to dreams that feel "active," like practicing a sport or running from something.

The limbic system: This is where we process our emotions, and it's most active during REM sleep — the reason why REM dreams tend to feel more expressive than those from other stages.

Lucid Dreaming

Normally when we dream, we're not actually aware that we're dreaming. So we go along for the ride with whatever bizarre scenarios our brain comes up with for us. But when more of our brain gets in on the fun (namely the parts that are related to higher cognitive function, attention, working memory, planning, and self-consciousness), things get a little more . . . real. Suddenly we're aware that we're in a dream and, with the same cognitive abilities we have in real life, can even control what happens and what we do. This is called lucid dreaming.

Lucid dreaming gets less and less frequent the older we get (it drops off pretty steeply after age 25), but a small percentage of people (about 20 percent) experience lucid dreams at least once a month. And it's estimated that about 50 percent of us have had at least one lucid dream in our lifetime.[75]

It's not clear what purpose lucid dreaming serves, nor do we really know why some people lucid dream more than others. It's suspected that certain neurochemicals may "switch on" parts of our consciousness when they would normally be switched off, so some people may just be naturally equipped with that neurochemical cocktail. Some researchers have found a connection between increased B6 intake and lucid dreaming,[76] while others have discovered associations between people who have strong moods, anxiety, and depression and those who have a higher frequency of lucid dreaming.[77] The ability to recall dreams in general is another predictor of lucid dreams, as is adopting a meditation practice—a 2015 study found that people who regularly practiced mindfulness were more likely to experience lucid dreams.[78]

Choose Your Own Adventure

One of the coolest features of lucid dreaming is that you can, in theory, learn how to do it—and then be a more active participant in your dreams. It's a way to explore activities that defy real-life logic (ever wanted to fly?), face your fears, or dig deeper into your subconscious. These are the most popular techniques used to harness your dream state:

1. Get better sleep. The more REM sleep you get, the longer and more vivid your dreams will be. And to get more REM, you need to be getting long stretches of deep, uninterrupted sleep.

2. Meditate. According to the aforementioned 2015 study, attention to the present state of consciousness while awake and contemplating whether the current experience might be a dream is one of the core techniques in a lucid dream practice.

3. Keep a dream journal. The most important step toward lucid dreaming is tuning into your dreams and recognizing that you're dreaming. The moment you wake up, write down anything and everything you remember from your dreams. Then revisit these details to look for patterns — what do you tend to dream about? As you're dreaming, you'll begin to be able to identify these "dream signs" and recognize that you're in a dream state.

4. Do a reality check. Lucid dreaming experts recommend doing frequent "reality checks" throughout the day to confirm whether you're awake or dreaming. When you're awake, it's obvious that you're not dreaming, but the repetition of these reality-affirming actions makes you more likely to repeat them when you're asleep. These are a few of the techniques, which experts recommend doing 10 times a day:

   - Reading a clock or a page of text, glancing away, and then looking back. In a dream, the time and text are likely to change.
   - Look at your hands and feet — they tend to be distorted in dreams.

- Try pushing the index finger of one hand through the palm of your opposite hand. Do it with the expectation that you'll be successful, and ask yourself whether you're dreaming. If you are successful, you'll know that you are, in fact, dreaming.

5. **Keep it MILD.** An acronym for Mnemonic Induction to Lucid Dreaming, the MILD technique is basically a self-awareness exercise for your brain. In this case, it's repeating a mantra along the lines of "I will know that I'm dreaming" or "I am dreaming" until you fall asleep.

6. **Go back to sleep.** Instead of immediately writing down a particularly vivid dream after you've woken up, try going back to sleep and re-entering the dream. But this time, be mindful of the fact that you are dreaming.

7. **Keep dreaming.** If you are successful in lucid dreaming, *staying* in the dream can be difficult at first. This can be because the realization that you're dreaming is so exciting that you get a jolt of adrenaline, or because you, oddly enough, forget you're dreaming. In order to settle into this new state, expert lucid dreamers recommend techniques for going deeper into your dream and essentially distracting your mind from waking up:

   - Do a simple math equation (e.g., "$3 + 3 = 6$"). Engaging a high-functioning part of your brain helps you build and keep consciousness while dreaming.
   - Rub your hands together or spin around. Research has found that initiating movement with your mind can stimulate the conscious brain further, drawing more awareness to your dream state body.
   - Stay calm. Getting overexcited or alarmed will cause a dream to end abruptly. Lucid dream experts suggest looking at your hands in order to center yourself in the moment.

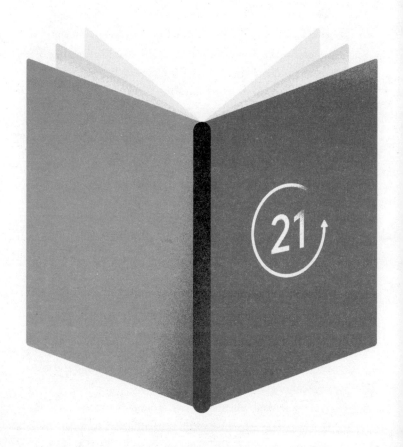

CHAPTER 10

THE RESET

Hi, Sleepy Person!

We developed this reset to help you supercharge your sleep, leave you feeling ready to take on the day, and make you actually excited to hop into bed at night. We've even put it to the test for you, making sure that it's as helpful as possible. As part of Casper's Sleep Advisory Board, Frank came to educate the Casper team about what goes into a good night's sleep and how they themselves can do better in the z's department. He challenged them to undertake a 21-day recalibration reset of their sleep habits, logging which habits worked and which didn't along the way. Not surprisingly, people who for years had struggled with their sleep were feeling refreshed and rested. Coffee addicts were reformed, night owls returned to their original lark rhythm, and pretty much everyone was logging less screen time in the p.m. Every week, small groups of the participants made a point of catching up, comparing notes, and cheering one another on. And after three weeks, we reconvened to share everyone's findings, fine-tuned the program, and The Reset was officially born.

So let's turn those yawns into smiles!

Over the next three weeks (or 21 days, if that makes you feel better), you're going to start shifting your rhythm, kicking the habits that steal from your sleep, and adding new habits that will help you cruise through the snooze. Along the way, we'll have you chart your results and feedback so that you can become your very own sleep scientist, gathering data about what's working and what's not. Because if there's one thing that can stand guard against late-night snacking or scrolling through your feed at 11 p.m., it's cold, hard facts. Also, you'll know whether a habit is useful for you, or not. When the three weeks are over, we encourage you to revisit your not-sleeping type (page 45) in order to further tailor your sleep-better protocol to your unique needs.

Because we want to set you up for success, we also highly recommend that you create a support system for yourself, whether it's one friend or a group. This will not only hold you accountable and provide some powerful motivation, but it will also make the experience as fun and enjoyable as sleep should be. Think of it as a new kind of book club! The folks at Casper loved knowing that they were in it together, helping each other troubleshoot, and sharing their victories.

A week before you start The Reset, have a kick-off meeting to make sure everyone knows the plan, and maybe share some of your hopes and fears about the next 21 days. Every week, pick a day to do a quick 15-minute check-in, whether it's a phone call, video chat, or text thread. After the final week, have a debrief about what worked, what you each would like to keep up with, and commitments that you want help sticking to. Then treat yourself to a nice, long, restful night's sleep.

Sleep well!

GOAL:

Prioritize your body's natural rhythm by making small changes to your habits.

ADJUSTMENTS:

1 Create a consistent schedule for getting to bed and waking up — make sure it allows for getting the sleep you need! (At least seven hours.)

2 Create a consistent mealtime schedule based on our recommendations on page 138. (We'll be tweaking the timing in Week 2 — for now, just stay consistent.)

3 Let sunshine into your room before checking texts and answering emails. (Bonus: Aim to get natural sun exposure throughout the day, even if it's just sitting by a window.)

4 Dim the lights and turn your electronics to "night mode" an hour and a half before bed.

GOAL:

Say goodbye to habits that have become barriers to healthy sleep.

ADJUSTMENTS:

1 Keep an eye on sugars and refined carbs throughout the day.

2 Say no to snacking, dinners, or alcohol at least an hour before bedtime.

3 Skip caffeine runs after 11 a.m.

4 No screens one hour before bed.

5 Block out unnecessary light from your bedroom.

GOAL:

Develop new healthy habits that create lasting change.

ADJUSTMENTS:

1 Add gut-healing measures to your meals (take a prebiotic, eat probiotic foods, get more leafy greens on your plate, steer clear of biome-bombing glyphosate).

2 Make lunch the biggest meal of the day.

3 Add one sanctuary-making touch to your bedroom.

4 Add one powering-down practice like stretching, deep breathing, or taking a warm bath.

ACKNOWLEDGMENTS

We would like to send our heartfelt thanks and gratitude to those who made this book possible:

From Frank:
To my young brother and intellectually curious co-writer Neil Parikh, whose passion for helping people sleep better inspired me to take on this project with him.

To our thoughtful, insightful, thorough co-writer Rachel Holtzman, who managed to take our information and complicated concepts and write a user-friendly, practical book.

To my longtime book agent, Stephanie Tade, whose support, guidance, and friendship never waver.

To the team at Little, Brown, including Marissa Vigilante and Ian Straus for their enthusiasm, patience, and attention to detail.

To my staff at the Eleven Eleven Wellness Center, in particular Vicky Zodo, who takes such good care of me, the practice, and all our patients. And to our nutritionist Dawn Brighid for supporting our patients on their health journeys and supporting me in getting a clear message out to the world.

To my daughter, Alison, son-in-law Zach, and grandson Benjamin, for bringing such joy into our lives.

To my incredible wife, Janice, who for more than forty years has put up with me, supported me, fed me, loved me, and been my greatest ally.

And finally to my patients, who constantly teach me and inspire me to find ways to make the world a happier and healthier place for all.

From Neil:

To my doctor, mentor, and older brother Frank, who opened a whole new world to me and thought of the idea for this book while putting needles in my back.

To our amazing co-author Rachel, whose incredible ability to make complicated subjects easily accessible made this book (and our journey writing it together) so much fun.

To my grandparents, who made the brave journey to the United States and inspired me to think big.

To my parents, for believing in me and supporting all of my endeavors.

To my loving wife, Sarah, whose positivity and generous heart motivates me to be better every day.

To my friends, new and old, for making life a great adventure.

To my co-founders at Casper, Luke, Gabe, Jeff, and Philip, for taking a chance on one another and for being great partners and friends on the ride of a lifetime.

To our current and former Casper team, who showed up every day to build something even bigger than a company—and, most importantly, became great friends along the way.

To Casper, who showed that a simple idea could help the world rest a little more.

NOTES

1. https://neurosciencenews.com/sleep-deprivation-genetics-10638/
2. https://www.ncbi.nlm.nih.gov/pmc/articles/PMC2276139/
3. https://www.sciencedaily.com/releases/2019/10/191002075944.htm
4. https://aaafoundation.org/acute-sleep-deprivation-risk-motor-vehicle-crash-involvement/
5. https://www.sleepfoundation.org/excessive-sleepiness/safety/relationship-between-sleep-and-industrial-accidents
6. https://www.sciencedirect.com/science/article/pii/S0733861917300245
7. https://www.ncbi.nlm.nih.gov/pubmed/25028798
8. https://www.sciencealert.com/deep-sleep-is-the-anti-anxiety-drug-we-ve-been-looking-for-brain-scans-reveal
9. https://www.futurity.org/sleep-loss-anger-1917812-2/
10. https://news.berkeley.edu/2018/08/14/sleep-viral-loneliness/
11. https://www.sciencedaily.com/releases/2019/02/190213132317.htm?utm_source=dlvr.it&utm_medium=twitter
12. https://newatlas.com/poor-sleep-heart-disease/58939/
13. https://www.outsideonline.com/2292806/your-body-no-sleep
14. https://medicalxpress.com/news/2020-03-irregular-cardiovascular-events.html
15. https://www.medicaldaily.com/poor-sleep-may-weaken-mens-fertility-402022
16. https://news.berkeley.edu/2013/08/06/poor-sleep-junk-food/
17. https://www.webmd.com/diet/obesity/video/obesity-risks
18. https://www.ncbi.nlm.nih.gov/pmc/articles/PMC3768102/
19. https://medicalxpress.com/news/2020-08-memories.html
20. https://www.nbcnews.com/better/health/what-happens-your-body-brain-while-you-sleep-ncna805276
21. https://articles.mercola.com/sites/articles/archive/2013/10/31/sleep-brain-detoxification.aspx
22. https://www.ncbi.nlm.nih.gov/pmc/articles/PMC3921176/
23. https://www.sciencedaily.com/releases/2019/03/190305170106.htm
24. https://www.ncbi.nlm.nih.gov/pmc/articles/PMC2913764/
25. https://pubmed.ncbi.nlm.nih.gov/25402367/
26. https://academic.oup.com/jcem/article/90/8/4530/3058888
27. https://sanescohealth.com/blog/10-things-your-body-does-while-you-sleep/
28. https://www.consumerreports.org/drugs/the-problem-with-sleeping-pills/

29. https://aasm.org/resources/pdf/pharmacologictreatmentofinsomnia.pdf
30. https://aasm.org/resources/pdf/pharmacologictreatmentofinsomnia.pdf
31. https://www.consumerreports.org/drugs/the-problem-with-sleeping-pills/
32. https://www.ncbi.nlm.nih.gov/pmc/articles/PMC4504291/pdf/AJPH.2015.302723.pdf
33. https://www.consumerreports.org/drugs/the-problem-with-sleeping-pills/
34. https://www.everydayhealth.com/sleep/1119/sleeping-pill-linked-to-hospital-falls.aspx
35. https://www.rxlist.com/benzodiazepines/drug-class.htm
36. https://www.drugabuse.gov/drugs-abuse/opioids/benzodiazepines-opioids
37. https://www.ncbi.nlm.nih.gov/pmc/articles/PMC4816010/
38. https://www.drugabuse.gov/drugs-abuse/opioids/benzodiazepines-opioids
39. https://www.scientificamerican.com/podcast/episode/weekday-weekend-sleep-imbalance-bad-for-blood-sugar-regulation/
40. https://www.ncbi.nlm.nih.gov/pubmed/23910656
41. https://www.nature.com/articles/s41598-018-36791-5
42. https://www.sleephealthjournal.org/article/S2352-7218(17)30041-4/fulltext
43. https://www.ncbi.nlm.nih.gov/pmc/articles/PMC4378297/
44. https://www.ncbi.nlm.nih.gov/pmc/articles/PMC3265077/
45. https://www.theatlantic.com/health/archive/2012/03/your-bodys-internal-clock-and-how-it-affects-your-overall-health/254518/
46. https://www.ncbi.nlm.nih.gov/pmc/articles/PMC4008810/#CR31
47. https://www.sciencedirect.com/science/article/abs/pii/S2352721819301056?via%3Dihub
48. https://libres.uncg.edu/ir/asu/listing.aspx?id=8000
49. https://www.ncbi.nlm.nih.gov/pmc/articles/PMC3077056/
50. https://www.ncbi.nlm.nih.gov/pubmed/31589627
51. https://www.ncbi.nlm.nih.gov/pmc/articles/PMC6290721/
52. https://jcsm.aasm.org/doi/10.5664/jcsm.5384
53. https://www.nhlbi.nih.gov/news/2019/added-sugars-refined-carbs-linked-insomnia-postmenopausal-women
54. https://www.sciencedaily.com/releases/2020/01/200103111717.htm
55. https://journals.physiology.org/doi/abs/10.1152/jappl.1956.8.5.556
56. https://www.ncbi.nlm.nih.gov/pubmed/17612945
57. https://www.sciencedaily.com/releases/2009/09/090901082552.htm
58. https://medicalxpress.com/news/2019-10-commonly-drugs-profoundly-affecting-gut.html
59. https://www.sleepfoundation.org/articles/how-medications-may-affect-sleep
60. https://www.ncbi.nlm.nih.gov/pmc/articles/PMC6213953/
61. https://onlinelibrary.wiley.com/doi/full/10.1111/j.1479-8425.2007.00262.x
62. https://www.ncbi.nlm.nih.gov/pubmed/22738673
63. https://www.sciencedaily.com/releases/2020/02/200203104505.htm
64. http://www.5gappeal.eu/about/
65. https://www.sleep.org/articles/aging-need-less-sleep/
66. https://www.ncbi.nlm.nih.gov/pubmed?cmd=search
67. https://www.sciencedaily.com/releases/2019/10/191001083956.htm

68. https://www.ncbi.nlm.nih.gov/pmc/articles/PMC2802254/

69. https://www.eurekalert.org/pub_releases/2019-05/esoe-spi051519.php

70. https://www.cdc.gov/features/students-sleep/index.html

71. https://www.aadsm.org/teen_drowsy_driving.php

72. https://www.ncbi.nlm.nih.gov/pmc/articles/PMC3079906/

73. https://www.psychologytoday.com/us/blog/dream-factory/201805/more-evidence
-dreams-reflect-learning-during-sleep

74. https://www.ncbi.nlm.nih.gov/pmc/articles/PMC3768102/

75. https://www.medicalnewstoday.com/articles/326496#How-common-are-lucid
-dreams?

76. https://www.medicalnewstoday.com/articles/326496#The-role-of-diet-and
-meditation

77. https://www.medicalnewstoday.com/articles/326496#How-common-are-lucid
-dreams?

78. https://journals.sagepub.com/doi/abs/10.1177/0276236615572594?journalCode
=icaa&

INDEX

ABOUT THE AUTHORS

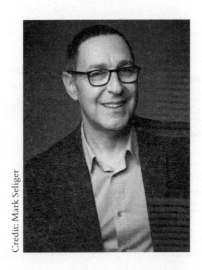

Credit: Mark Seliger

Frank Lipman, MD, is a pioneer and internationally recognized expert in the fields of Integrative and Functional Medicine, as well as the founder and director of Eleven Eleven Wellness Center in New York City, one of the best-known Integrative Medicine centers in the country. Frank is a *New York Times* bestselling author who is dedicated to simplifying a whole-systems approach to optimal health for today's reader. His most recent books, *The New Health Rules* and *How to Be Well,* broke the mold of health books by offering a dynamic and user-friendly guide to building better health one step at a time. It succeeded in reaching beyond the health-book audience and into a broad general public, perfectly setting the stage for *Sleep Well*.

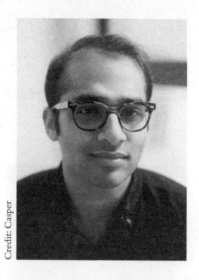

Credit: Casper

Neil Parikh is the Co-founder and Chief Strategy Officer at Casper, the world's first sleep brand that dominates global e-commerce in addition to having twenty Sleep Shops across North America and selling at retailers such as Target and Hudson's Bay. Casper has sold mattresses to over a million consumers, with sales topping $400 million in 2018. This year, Casper officially joined the unicorn club, with a valuation exceeding $1 billion. As the son of a sleep doctor, Neil has been perfectly positioned to bridge the gap between the science of sleep and the realities of the sleep industry. He was accepted to medical school at seventeen, worked on robotics at NASA (where he co-authored 3 patents), and in 2014 launched Casper.

Rachel Holtzman is a bestselling co-author who has written over thirty books on topics ranging from wellness and mind-body connection, to cooking and entertaining, to personal growth and inspiration. Prior to working as a collaborator, she was an editor at Penguin Books and ELLE magazine, with a brief turn in the kitchen at Gramercy Tavern. She lives in Saint Louis.